Activity Techniques

Activity Techniques

That Heal the Wounds of Alzheimer's

Amira Choukair Tame, A.C.C.

To order additional copies of this book, contact:
Xlibris Corporation
1-888-795-4274
www.Xlibris.com
Orders@Xlibris.com
46891

Contents

Acknowledgments/Introduction

Working with Alzheimer's has given me a deep respect for the caregivers and professionals who work every day to help alleviate the symptoms of this devastating disease.

I thank the Alzheimer's Association for helping us understand what Alzheimer's disease is about and for providing those in need with compassion, support and resourceful guidance.

I thank my peers and other professionals who encouraged me to write this second edition.

Thanks to Mike Akra of DocuMall for his painstaking effort to present my material in a way that is informative and easy to read.

Also, I want to thank Mary Shoucair for her literary and grammatical guidance.

Last, but not least, I thank my loving husband for years of patience and encouragement that helped make this dream come true.

And in the end
It's not the years
In your life that count
It's the life in your years
—Abraham Lincoln

"Amira, your work really touches people and moves them. You inspire others to action."

Steve Wilson,
Founder, President and Cheerman of The Bored (tm)
World Laughter Tour, Inc. www.WorldLaughterTour.com

About the Author

Amira is an energetic Activities Professional, with many years of experience, who is dedicated to the advancement of non-drug therapy for persons with Alzheimer's disease and other dementia disorders. Providing therapeutic activities for hundreds of people suffering with Alzheimer's disease has given her an opportunity to develop activities that are successful at any stage of dementia. Amira has shared her techniques with other professionals through caregiver training sessions and workshops. Training Hospice care volunteers has been especially rewarding.

Amira is a Nationally Certified Activities Consultant (NCCAP) and a member of the Michigan Association of Activities Professionals, the National Association of Activities Professionals, and a member of the Alzheimer Association. Her techniques have gained the trust and respect of her peers, the medical community, and most importantly, those she has helped to re-establish a sense of respect and dignity to their lives — the person with Alzheimer's disease.

From the Author

When I started working in a facility that cared for residents with Alzheimer's disease, I already had several years experience working with the elderly and mentally impaired, so I was confident of my ability to improve their quality of life, but I soon realized I had much to learn.

My first day at the nursing home was very frustrating. I confidently brought various materials with me and arranged them on the table in the activity room. The table had chairs strategically placed around it. All I needed to do was lead the residents to the table and seat them. Then we could proceed with my planned activities. Right? Wrong!

I brought a few residents to the table, seated them, and went back for the rest. When I returned to the activity room with the second group, I found the first group had left. That first day's allotted two hours of activity time was spent playing hide and seek and the residents actively eluding me.

When I began working with residents in various stages of Alzheimer's, it didn't take long for me to realize that for my activities to be successful I had to address the fear, anger, frustration, low self-esteem, and other negative feelings that were barriers to success. I felt confident that I could help return some of the residents' memory function and teach them new activities if I got to know them and their likes and dislikes.

I soon recognized that Alzheimer's residents had their own set of issues and needs and I would have to customize my repertoire of activities to accommodate those issues and needs. Not only did I recognize a need for specialized activities for residents with Alzheimer's, I realized that because of the progressive nature of Alzheimer's disease, activities had to be easily adjusted to each individual's abilities and needs and closely monitored to keep in sync with those abilities.

I spent the next several months studying the behavioral effects of Alzheimer's disease and searching for activities that could be modified to the changing abilities of my residents. What seemed to be missing from the information I read was any hope that abilities or memory functions could be improved. This did not seem to be reasonable to me because I already knew that I made a difference with elderly persons using my activities for many years. I decided to try the same activities modified for Alzheimer's residents.

To my delight, I was not only able to introduce new activities to my residents, I was seeing improvements in memory function and return of self-confidence. What was I doing that made me so successful? I began to keep a log of what worked with some residents and what did not with others. The successful combination of the methods, techniques and activities inspired me to write this book. I felt compelled to share

Amira C. Tame, A.C.C.

my success with others. I did not want my book to be another technical manual with difficult-to-read rules and regulations or a long list of activities without explanation of how to be successful with them. What I did want was to provide a guide that could help you achieve the success that I've had with my Alzheimer's clients; for the professional, a supplement to the well-established procedures and documentation guidelines. And for the person caring for someone at home, an easy to read, comprehensive guide to healing the wounds of Alzheimer's disease.

Testimonials

From caregivers

"Dear Amira,

I remember when I called you, and we talked about my wife's Alzheimer's disease and her difficulty to remember things, and her anger at me, and the argument with no reason. Your positive conversation helped me to hire you to help my wife to reduce her anger and stimulate her mind, and I asked you to see my wife two times a week. Well let me tell you my wife she said she needs no body around, but you really made a difference with my wife. She liked you and amazingly she liked to participate in the activities and she liked to do things, because you gave a reason to help you as a volunteer, I really realize how much you could make a difference for my wife but always there's some good days and some bad days. *Amira I am glad I met you, you helped my wife in many ways.*

—Lester

"To whom it may concern,

I have known Amira Tame for one and a half years. We employed her when my mother first moved into a senior apartment and she was very agitated and unhappy. Amira has proven to be a big help in my mother's case. My mother at first was not too comfortable with strangers, but over time she came to trust Amira and enjoyed her company. She now feels secure in her presence. My mother's short term memory is very poor, but when she sees Amy, I feel she considers her a friend.

Amira has tried to vary her activities and has taken my mother out of the facility for a ride and has included a lot of the other residents at times. The American house has now employed her due to her rapport with these people. We have been very satisfied with Amira's assistance and friendship with my mother"

—Corinne

Amira C. Tame, A.C.C.

September 3, 2004

Dear Amira,

You may be pleased to know how much I have appreciated your work with my sister, Adela Valverde.

Her eyes would sparkle with joy as you entered the room and greeted her.

Throughout the last six years of her life she responded enthusiastically to your suggestions — inter-acting with you to the best of her ever-diminishing ability in various projects and games. Your skill and patience brought out the best in her.

Also — thank you for the video you made of your last session with her — one day before she slipped out of consciousness on her 10-day slide to death.

Sincerely,
Mary S Foucair

Dear Amira I Enjoy Being with you I like to be your today is thursday 1994 Sincerely

1) If you think you need help ask Amira. She can help you because She Have talken with her Work. ACTIVITTES

Dorit → 3/28/1996

Esther

Amira
1. is a very nice girl.
She is always Kind to Me.
3. She is very nice. because She tries to help other people,

3/28/1996

Esther Gordon

Dorit

Amira Chavoushair
Dear Amira I like you very
Much
You are a very nice person you Smile
all the time

You Make Me feel better
when you are around.
My Name is Esther
Today is Monday

"Mrs. Choukair has a gentle manner when dealing with those in our society who suffer with the symptoms of Alzheimer's disease. I have witnessed her work personally and appreciate her ability to reach inside those who seem unreachable and her talent at bringing out whatever parts have been hidden by this devastating disease".

—Victoria Kowaleski
Publisher of Caregiver monthly newsletter

"Amira Tame, Program Trainer for Alzheimer Activities Unit, is a professional, energetic and caring person. She has an excellent understanding of the emotional and social needs of seniors. Our residents always enjoy the time spent with her".

—J. Robert Gillette—President
American House Retirement Residences

"While I was participating in the Alzheimer's Activities Workshop on March 24, 2005, I observed how each person was reacting to the techniques that Amira was showing them. I encouraged one of our residents, Mary, to participate. Mary has a hearing and speech impairment and dementia. Mary sits for hours a day smiling and never participates in our activities. During this particular activity we were singing "You Are My Sunshine." Mary was watching as everyone was singing. I noticed that she was watching Amira and she began to sing the song with us. This was a tremendous accomplishment. Amira definitely has the skill to reach inside a senior citizen and bring out their inner feelings and talents. I was impressed with the workshop and found Amira's advice to be very beneficial.

—Marie Tester
Activities Director
Maple Heights Retirement Community

" . . . . Most directly, one of our CLLs is an expert on activities for Alzheimer's patients. She is Amira Choukair Tame, and is the author of "Healing the Wounds of Alzheimer's." She has a new book and excellent instructional CD, "The ABC's of Activites for Alzheimer's." Amira was one of the outstanding presenters at this year's Advanced CLL Workshop." "Amira's books and CD are 'must-have' resources for everyone who cares about a person with Alzheimer's. Her methods can be understood and used effectively by almost anybody at any level, professionals, volunteers, friends, and family members, too."

Steve Wilson,
Founder, President and Cheerman of The Bored(tm)
World Laughter Tour, Inc. www.WorldLaughterTour.com

"Amira, your work really touches people and moves them. You inspire others to action."

Steve Wilson

A few weeks ago, in Columbus, Ohio, I was privileged to attend an Alzheimer's Presentation produced by Amira Choukair Tame. As part of the program, Amira played a DVD called "The ABC's of Alzheimer's."

The DVD was a masterpiece of education depicting the activities, the humanism of the care giver, the spontaneous actions resulting in the professional way the care giver in a most un-pressured manner was able to secure reactions from the patient. Explanation of the individual activities to be performed was followed by actual demonstrations of the wonderful un-pressured responses by the patient to the care giver. The DVD included a great variety of situations and activities to be performed. The program followed the progress of the patients, right up to a sensational climax on the final days of life. To reveal the last two minutes of the program on paper would not do justice to the most wonderful conclusion of any real life situation I have ever had the privilege of viewing.

To all care givers, friends, relatives of anyone who is afflicted with Alzheimer's, the book, and "The ABC's of Alzheimer's" are a joy, full of human kindness, and a wonderful prescription for those who care. It has my heartiest recommendation.

Most respectfully submitted,
Bob Butler

Introduction

Although Alzheimer's is a progressive and irreversible disease, I've found that through proper application of therapeutic activities the progression of behavioral effects caused by memory decline can be delayed and, in some cases, reversed.

Implementing an activities program for residents with Alzheimer's is usually a challenging and difficult task. Often there are barriers of mistrust, fear, anxiety, low self-esteem and self-confidence, resentment and confusion that must be overcome. Even the most caring attempts to be helpful or to communicate are sometimes met with outbursts of anger, resistance, or complete withdrawal. With my approach, I believe that activity therapy can reduce the negative behavioral effects caused by Alzheimer's disease, and have a positive effect on memory function.

My common-sense approach in utilizing the practical and logical therapeutic activities described in this book can be easily adopted and enhanced to improve the quality of life for those affected by Alzheimer's disease. Each approach is tailored to individual needs by utilizing whatever mental and physical skills the person still possesses and, furthermore, continuously enhancing these skills.

It's not enough to love and care for someone and want them to get better. It takes strong determination to learn as much as possible about Alzheimer's disease, believe in your ability to make a significant improvement, and have enough patience and dedication to achieve positive results.

Sometimes the only way to deal with stress is to find humor in one's situation.

When it comes to dealing with Alzheimer's disease, a smile often works better than words. Humor and light-heartedness are often the best medicine for the stress the disease brings to you and the person you're caring for.

Who Can Benefit?

Whether you utilize the services of an Alzheimer therapist or shoulder the burden yourself, this book is essential in providing the most appropriate caregiving plan, including helping you select the most effective caregiver for your loved one. This book provides easy to understand and apply activities utilizing readily available materials. Seventy percent of the 4 million Americans with Alzheimer's disease are cared for at home.

Caregivers providing care for their loved one at home

This book is written to be used by the caregiver who does not have a professional caregiving background. The documentation forms are designed to assist you in collecting useful data about the individual you are caring for, without burdening you with complex guidelines for professional caregivers.
Furthermore, when considering residential care, you will know how to assess the treatment program and gain understanding of the basics of a successful activities program.

Friends and Family Members

I would advise anyone who plans to visit regularly to read this book so they can help contribute to the success of your activities program. It will even help occasional visitors spend quality time when visiting. The activity program provides guidelines to successful communication skills and techniques that help repair your relationship with the person you're caring for. Understanding the concepts, tools and techniques will make you feel more comfortable visiting a friend or relative with Alzheimer's disease.

Amira C. Tame, A.C.C.

Professional caregivers

As a professional caregiver, you will gain insight by reading actual case studies on how I work with my clients. You will learn new methodologies and concepts that have worked with hundreds of persons in all stages of the disease. Understanding the principles behind the design of these activities will complement and add to your own techniques, tools and activities.
As you read through the chapters of this book, you will be reminded of how important it is to show respect and love to the person suffering from this disease.

- **When we bring sunshine into lives of others, we are warmed by it ourselves.**
- **Walk through the light and darkness of their experience.**
- **We must take care of our children for they have a long way to go.**
- **We must take care of the elders for they have come a long way.**
- **We must take care of the in-between for they are doing much work.**
- **Listen completely to their stories; they need to be told.**
- **When an elder dies it is as if a library has burned.**
- **A person is only dead when no one calls their name.**
- **When we stand tall, we are standing on the shoulders of our ancestors.**

Chapter 1

Understanding Alzheimer's Disease and Its Devastating Effects

Life's Journey

Do not set your goals by what other people deem important.

Only you know what is best for you.

Do not take for granted the things closest to your heart.

Cling to them as you would your life, for without them, life is meaningless.

Do not let your life slip through your fingers by living in the past nor for the future.

By living your life one day at a time, you live all of the days of your life.

Do not give up when you still have something to give.

To be without hope is to be without purpose.

Nothing is really over until the moment you stop trying.

It is a fragile thread that binds us to each other.

Do not shut love out of your life.

The quickest way to receive love is to give love.

Amira C. Tame, A.C.C.

Understanding the Changes

When I began to compile information for this book several years ago, I came across this article authored by Tim Brennan. His account of how Alzheimer's disease had impacted his life was so eloquent. I truly felt I could not have said it any better. Many people with Alzheimer's and their caregivers have had similar experiences.

Excerpts from an article written by Tim Brennan in the *Detroit News*, March 26, 1995.

Sixteen months ago, I was diagnosed as having Alzheimer's disease.

Prior to the diagnosis, my wife and I went from one doctor to another, searching for answers to the mind-related problems I was experiencing. During this search, frequently I would ask myself: "Are you crazy or what?"

During the early onset of Alzheimer's, it is extremely difficult for a doctor to properly diagnose the disease. It is also hard for the person to describe all the symptoms he or she may be experiencing, because we don't know what to look for to tell the doctor.

If you have the flu, often you will tell the doctor about the accompanying cold, chills and fever. The dementia problems I initially experienced included forgetfulness, errors with simple math, misspelling and mispronunciation of words once commonly used and loss of balance, among other difficulties. I don't know if I told the doctor of all the symptoms I was having at the time. I just thought I was probably crazy.

It was not easy to accept the doctor saying: "You have Alzheimer's disease." My wife and I cried and held each other for a long time following this revelation.

You see, there is no cure for this disease. No miracle drugs are available to stop or slow down its progress. No operation can be scheduled to cut out the parts, helping to heal the good ones that are left.

We both knew, without a word being spoken, that the doctor had just given me a death sentence, with no possibility of a last-minute reprieve.

For a while after the diagnosis, I had to tell myself I had Alzheimer's quite often in order to accept the fact my life had to change. Like the opening line from an AA meeting: "Hello, my name is Joe and I am an alcoholic," the first step toward making necessary life-style changes were, for me, to accept what I had as a problem or a condition. With Alzheimer's, I slowly learned and grew to accept change as being a necessary response to a gradually deteriorating brain.

At first, I learned I could no longer hold a full-time job. I love to work, and this change was difficult to accept. I then tried to put in a couple of hours a week of volunteer work and found out, each time, that it would take me a day and a half or more to recover mentally from the effort.

My mind was and is continuing to slowly leave me and each time something was lost, such as handwriting ability, shoelace tying or the memories of people and/or events, it set the stage for additional changes to be made with my life. Life is interactive.

Alzheimer's disease also required my wife to adjust her life to the changes in my life. As time went by, I could no longer grocery shop, so she assumed this duty. Eventually, she had to take over as the household finance manager and appointment maker. We no longer go to dances or to concerts together.

Whenever we are out together, she drives. The chores I am left to do around the house are simple and can be deferred, if necessary.

Our life is one of, more or less, constant change. My life has to be downsized each time further deterioration becomes evident and my wife adjusts to these changes with those required on her part. Things are much harder on my wife, who is my caregiver and mate for life. She sees the changes that Alzheimer's disease has brought about. She responds with love and understanding. Yet I know she has cried when no one else was nearby. She prays and I pray and this seems to help.

Amira C. Tame, A.C.C.

Our relationship is evolving. I am becoming more dependent. I don't want this to happen, but there is no choice. Slowly, I am becoming more of a child. My wife, in turn, makes more and more decisions about our life. We still interact, but my share of our adult relationship is gradually going away.

Still, there is much hope. As losses are incurred, I try to learn new things in order to keep the mind active. I play pool and shoot darts and write, often, to friends. I listen to novels on cassette tapes. Efforts are made to remember people's names. These activities help the mind function more capably.

Life is still good. It is now very different from what it once was. My life is very simple.

I'd like to offer some advice for those affected by Alzheimer's disease. To caregivers, I would say to keep on with love and affection as long as you possibly can. Don't let your health suffer because of the care you give to us. Seek out those who can help you with the burden our illness gives you. And when it is time for you to let us go, please do so without regret.

Place us in a nursing home or bury us and then hold your head up high. You gave us your best effort. There is nothing more to be done now. You must start over again with your own life.

To a person with Alzheimer's, the message is one of continuing to strive, to keep going forward no matter how difficult it may be. Ensure your family finances are in order before you lose the ability to make proper decisions in this area. Share a smile and laughter with all those you meet. Hug and kiss your loved ones. Keep your mind as active as possible, for this action will help you prolong or extend your mental life span. Live for today.

When I was lost, you showed the way.
When I was frightened, you calmed fear away.
You made me laugh, when I wanted to cry.
I fail so often and you tell me, "Just try."
You are my friend, and I forgot your name.
I called for help and it was you, who came . . .
The time is short and soon, I must go.
There's just one thing left for you to know.
The sun and rain help to make a garden grow.
The garden grew well, now winter threatens snow.
And so, I leave with a final loving refrain,
You are the sunshine—I am the rain.

—**Tim Brennan**

Amira C. Tame, A.C.C.

Do Tim's words sound familiar?
Do you feel his pain and suffering?
Does your life reflect any of the changes he described?
If so, this book will be your companion and guide to a more
fulfilling and happier life for you and the person you're caring for.

Facts about Alzheimer's Disease

Alzheimer's disease is a progressive, neurodegenerative disease characterized by memory loss, language deterioration, impaired visual-spatial skills, poor judgment, indifferent attitude, but preserved motor function. The term "Alzheimer's disease" is used to describe a dementing disorder marked by certain brain changes, regardless of the age of onset. Dementia causes a significant loss of intellectual abilities severe enough to interfere with social or occupational functioning. Dementia is not a disease in itself but a group of symptoms that may accompany certain diseases or physical conditions.

The cause and rate of progression of dementias vary. One of the most well-known diseases that produces dementia is Alzheimer's disease. Other conditions that may cause or mimic dementia include depression, brain tumors, nutritional deficiencies, head injuries, hydrocephalus, infections (AIDS, meningitis, syphilis), drug reactions and thyroid problems. It is highly recommended that all persons experiencing memory deficits or confusion undergo a thorough diagnostic evaluation. This requires examination by a physician experienced in the diagnosis of dementing disorders and detailed laboratory testing. The examination should include a re-evaluation of all medications. This process will help identify treatment for reversible conditions, aid the family in planning future care, and provide important medical information for future generations.

What Happens to the Brain?

How the Brain and Nerve Cells change during Alzheimer's disease

One of the hallmarks of Alzheimer's disease is the accumulation of amyloid plaques between nerve cells (neurons) in the brain. Amyloid is a general term for protein fragments that the body produces normally. Beta-amyloid is a fragment of a protein that is snipped from another protein called amyloid precursor protein (APP). In a healthy brain, these protein fragments would be broken down and eliminated. In Alzheimer's disease, the fragments accumulate to form hard, insoluble plaques. Neurofibrillary tangles consist of insoluble twisted fibers that are found inside of the brain's cells. They primarily consist of a protein called tau that forms part of a structure called a microtubule. The microtubule helps transport nutrients and other important substances from one part of the nerve cell to another. The axon is the long threadlike extension that conducts nerve impulses away from the body of a nerve cell, and dendrites are any of the short branched threadlike extensions that conduct nerve impulses towards the nerve cell body. In Alzheimer's disease the tau protein is abnormal and the microtubule structures collapse. There is an overall shrinkage of brain tissue as Alzheimer's disease progresses. In addition, the ventricles, or chambers within the brain that contain cerebrospinal fluid, are noticeably enlarged. In the early stages of Alzheimer's disease, short-term memory begins to decline when the cells in the hippocampus, that is part of the limbic system, degenerate. The ability to perform routine tasks also declines. As Alzheimer's disease spreads through the cerebral cortex (the outer layer of the brain), judgment declines, emotional outbursts may occur and language is impaired. Progression of the disease leads to the death of more nerve cells and subsequent behavior changes, such as wandering and agitation. The ability to recognize faces and to communicate is completely lost in the final stages. They eventually lose bowel and bladder control, and need constant care. This stage of complete dependency may last for years. The average length of time from diagnosis to death is 4 to 8 years, although it can take 20 years or more for the disease to run its course.

Recent Statistics

- Alzheimer's disease (AD) is a progressive, degenerative disease that attacks the brain and results in impaired memory, thinking and behavior, ultimately leaving them totally incapable of caring for themselves.
- Alzheimer's is the fourth leading cause of death in adults, claiming more than 100,000 lives annually. It affects males and females, ethnic and socioeconomic groups equally.
- Alzheimer's disease impacts 10% of the population over age 65 and up to 50% of those age 85 and older.

The aging of the population will continue to increase the number of individuals at risk.

The older population in the United States is dramatically increasing. As of the year 2000, an estimated 35 million people were age 65 and older. Researchers estimate that by 2050, 70 million Americans will be age 65 or older, accounting for 1 in 5 Americans. More than 19 million Americans will be age 85 and older.

- AD is the most common cause of dementia among people age 65 and older. Its current and future impact on our society can be seen in these few statistics:
- Scientists estimate that around 4.5 million people now have AD. For every 5-year age group beyond 65, the percentage of people with AD doubles.
- By 2050, 13.2 million older Americans are expected to have AD if the current numbers hold and no preventive treatments become available.
- Researchers recently projected the number of new cases of AD that could occur every year between 1995 and 2050. They estimate that the number will more than double—from 377,000 per year in 1995, to 959,000 per year in 2050.
- The annual number of new cases will increase sharply around 2040, when all baby boomers will be over 70.

Two factors will combine to cause this increase:

- The fact that AD risk increases as people get older.
- The growing numbers of older people, especially those over 85.

It appears that the number of AD cases may differ across racial and ethnic groups. Finding out more about this issue is an important focus of AD research.

Ten Warning Signs of Alzheimer's Disease

In most cases, one of the first manifestations is memory loss, having trouble remembering the familiar names, places, and facts of everyday life. After several years, cognition, personality, ability to function, judgment, concentration, orientation and speech are affected. During the latter stages of Alzheimer's, most lose all mental abilities as well as control over body functions.

To help you understand the warning signs to look for, the Alzheimer's Association has developed a checklist of common symptoms of

Amira C. Tame, A.C.C.

Alzheimer's disease (some symptoms may also apply to other dementing illnesses):

1. **RECENT MEMORY LOSS AFFECTING JOB SKILLS**
   It's normal to occasionally forget assignments, colleagues' names or a business associate's telephone number, and remember them later. Those with dementia, such as Alzheimer's disease, may forget things more often, and not remember them later. They repeatedly may ask the same question, not remembering the answer.

2. **DIFFICULTY PERFORMING FAMILIAR TASKS**
   Busy people can be so distracted from time to time that they may leave the carrots on the stove and only remember to serve them at the end of the meal. People with Alzheimer's disease could prepare a meal and not only forget to serve it, but also forget they made it.

3. **PROBLEMS WITH LANGUAGE**
   Everyone has trouble finding the right word sometimes but can finish the sentence with another appropriate word. A person with Alzheimer's disease may forget simple words, or substitute inappropriate words, making their sentence incomprehensible.

4. **DISORIENTATION OF TIME AND PLACE**
   It's normal to forget the day of the week or your destination for a moment. But people with Alzheimer's disease can become lost on their own street or in a familiar mall, not knowing where they are, how they got there or how to get back home.

5. **POOR OR DECREASED JUDGMENT**
   People can become so immersed in an activity or telephone conversation they temporarily forget the child they're watching.
   A person with Alzheimer's disease could forget the child under their care and leave the house to visit a neighbor. They may dress inappropriately, wearing several shirts or blouses.

6. **PROBLEMS WITH ABSTRACT THINKING**
   People who normally balance their checkbooks may be momentarily disconcerted when the task is more complicated than usual, but will eventually figure out the solution. Someone with Alzheimer's disease

could forget completely what the numbers are and what needs to be done with them.

7. MISPLACING THINGS
   Anyone can lose their wallet or keys, but eventually find them by reconstructing where they could have left them. A person with Alzheimer's disease may put things in inappropriate places: an iron in the freezer, or a wristwatch in the sugar bowl.

8. CHANGES IN MOOD OR BEHAVIOR
   Everyone has a bad day once in a while, or may become sad or moody from time to time. Someone with Alzheimer's disease can exhibit rapid mood swings for no apparent reason: e.g., from calm to tears to anger to calm within a few moments.

9. CHANGES IN PERSONALITY
   People's personalities ordinarily change somewhat at different ages, as character traits strengthen or mellow. But a person with Alzheimer's disease can change drastically, becoming extremely confused, irritable, suspicious or fearful.

10. LOSS OF INITIATIVE
    It's normal to tire of housework, business activities or social obligations, but most people regain their initiative. A person with Alzheimer's disease may become passive and require cues and prompting to get them involved in activities.

Understanding the Stages of Alzheimer's Disease

Over the years, numerous assessment scales have been used by physicians and other professionals in an attempt to identify the stages of Alzheimer's disease more clearly. The intent is to obtain as much information as possible about how the disease progresses in order to help families and professionals better understand specific care needs.

It is difficult to place a person with Alzheimer's disease in a specific stage. However, symptoms seem to progress in a recognizable pattern and these stages provide a framework for understanding the disease. It is important to remember they are not uniform in every instance and the stages often overlap.

Experts have documented common patterns of symptom progression that occur in many individuals with Alzheimer's disease, and developed several methods of "staging" based on these patterns. Progression of symptoms corresponds in a general way to the underlying nerve cell degeneration that takes place in Alzheimer's disease. Nerve cell damage typically begins with cells involved in learning and memory and gradually spreads to cells that control every aspect of thinking, judgment, and behavior. The damage eventually affects cells that control and coordinate movement.

Staging systems provide useful frames of reference for understanding how the disease may unfold and for making future plans. But it is important to note that all stages are artificial benchmarks in a continuous process that can vary greatly from one person to another. Not everyone will experience every symptom, and symptoms may occur at different times in different individuals. People with Alzheimer's live an average of 8 years after diagnosis, but may survive anywhere from 3 to 20 years.

The framework of this section is the Global Deterioration Scale, a system that outlines key symptoms characterizing seven stages ranging from unimpaired function to very severe cognitive decline.

Within this framework, we have noted which Global Deterioration Scale stages correspond to the widely used concepts of mild, moderate, moderately severe, and severe Alzheimer's disease. We have also noted which stages fall within the more general divisions of early-stage, mid-stage, and late-stage categories.

The Stages

First Stage

No cognitive impairment
Unimpaired individuals experience no memory problems and none are evident to a health care professional during a medical interview.

Second Stage

Very mild cognitive decline
Individuals at this stage feel as if they have memory lapses, especially in forgetting familiar words or names or the location of keys, eyeglasses, or other everyday objects. But these problems are not evident during a medical examination or apparent to friends, family, or co-workers.

Third Stage

Cognitive decline
Early-stage Alzheimer's can be diagnosed in some, but not all, individuals with these symptoms. Friends, family, or co-workers begin to notice deficiencies. Problems with memory or concentration may be measurable in clinical testing or discernible during a detailed medical interview. Common difficulties include:

- Word—or name-finding problems noticeable to family or close associates
- Decreased ability to remember names when introduced to new people
- Performance issues in social or work settings noticeable to family, friends, or co-workers
- Reading a passage and retaining little material
- Losing or misplacing a valuable object
- Decline in ability to plan or organize
- Complete disorientation to time and place
- Complete dependence
- Development of various forms of speech impairment

Amira C. Tame, A.C.C.

- Develop a need to put foreign objects into mouth and a need to touch everything

Fourth Stage

Moderate cognitive decline (Mild or early-stage Alzheimer's disease)
At this stage, a careful medical interview detects clear-cut deficiencies in the following areas:

- Decreased knowledge of recent occasions or current events
- Impaired ability to perform challenging mental arithmetic-for example, to count backward from 100 by 7s
- Decreased capacity to perform complex tasks, such as marketing, planning dinner for guests, or paying bills and managing finances. Reduced memory of personal history
- The affected individual may seem subdued and withdrawn, especially in socially or mentally challenging situations

Fifth Stage

Moderately severe cognitive decline (Moderate or mid-stage Alzheimer's disease)
Major gaps in memory and deficits in cognitive function emerge. Some assistance with day-to-day activities becomes essential. At this stage, individuals may:

- Be unable during a medical interview to recall such important details as their current address, their telephone number, or the name of the college or high school from which they graduated
- Become confused about where they are or about the date, day of the week, or season
- Have trouble with less challenging mental arithmetic; for example, counting backward from 40 by 4s or from 20 by 2s
- Need help choosing proper clothing for the season or the occasion
- Usually retain substantial knowledge about themselves and know their own name and the names of their spouse or children
- Usually require no assistance with eating or using the toilet

Sixth Stage

Severe cognitive decline (Moderately severe or mid-stage Alzheimer's disease)
Memory difficulties continue to worsen, significant personality changes may emerge, and affected individuals need extensive help with customary daily activities. At this stage, individuals may:

- Lose most awareness of recent experiences and events as well as their surroundings
- Recollect their personal history imperfectly, although they generally recall their own name
- Occasionally forget the name of their spouse or primary caregiver but generally can distinguish familiar from unfamiliar faces
- Need help getting dressed properly; without supervision, may make such errors as putting pajamas over daytime clothes or shoes on wrong feet
- Experience disruption of their normal sleep/waking cycle
- Need help with handling details of toileting (flushing toilet, wiping, and disposing of tissue properly)
- Have increasing episodes of urinary or fecal incontinence
- Experience significant personality changes and behavioral symptoms, including suspiciousness and delusions (for example, believing that their caregiver is an impostor); hallucinations (seeing or hearing things that are not really there); or compulsive, repetitive behaviors such as hand-wringing or tissue shredding
- Tend to wander and become lost

Seventh Stage

Very severe cognitive decline (Severe or late-stage Alzheimer's disease)
This is the final stage of the disease when individuals lose the ability to respond to their environment, the ability to speak, and, ultimately, the ability to control movement.

- Frequently individuals lose their capacity for recognizable speech, although words or phrases may occasionally be uttered
- Individuals need help with eating, exercise no control over elimination needs, and require periodic diaper changes

Amira C. Tame, A.C.C.

- Individuals lose the ability to walk without assistance, then the ability to sit without support, the ability to smile, and the ability to hold their head up. Reflexes become abnormal and muscles grow rigid
- Swallowing is impaired

Family/Caregiver Education and Support Services

Counseling and support are available through local chapters of the Alzheimer's Association, or through recommendations from a family physician, nurse, social worker, or other health care provider. Family members who are familiar with the behavioral symptoms of Alzheimer's and know how to effectively communicate with their loved one can better cope with challenging behaviors that develop as the disease progresses. Educational and emotional support can directly benefit families affected by Alzheimer's disease and may even delay a loved one's entry into a nursing home. With help and support throughout the disease process, families are able to take more control over their lives and make more informed decisions. Perhaps one of the greatest costs of AD is the physical and emotional toll on family, caregivers, and friends. Changes in the loved one and the constant caregiving duties can be both hard to bear and rewarding.

Research on caregiver support is still in the early stages. Even so, we've already learned a lot about the unique aspects of caregiving and needs for support.

Most primary caregivers are family members

- Not surprisingly, spouses are the largest group of caregivers. Most are older and may be dealing with their own health problems in addition to caring for the person with AD.
- Daughters are the second largest group of caregivers. Many have families of their own. Juggling two sets of responsibilities can be hard for these members of the "sandwich" generation.
- Sons and daughters-in-law also frequently shoulder caregiving responsibilities.
- Other family members, too, are involved. Brothers, sisters, and grandchildren may have unique needs for caregiving support.

Many other people participate in the care of those with AD. Friends, neighbors, work colleagues, and faith community members often help to care for the person with AD. They also play essential roles in supporting the primary caregivers. Studies have shown that caregivers of people with AD and other dementias spend significantly more time on caregiving tasks than do caregivers of people with other diseases. These studies also show that caregiving imposes a significant psychological and physical burden on families. Peer support programs that link caregivers with trained volunteers can help. Other research has confirmed that the information and problem-solving needs of caregivers evolve over time as the person with AD changes. Support programs can respond by offering services and information geared to the different stages of AD.

Support groups have always been an important feature of AD caregiver programs. But these groups have drawbacks. The participant must arrange care for the person with AD. The timing of the group may not coincide with the time that the participant needs advice or wants to express feelings. Some people are uncomfortable sharing in a public setting. Members of certain ethnic groups may be especially reluctant to join a support group. Fortunately, help is on the way. In one of the most exciting new areas of research, investigators are exploring ways to harness the power of the Internet to help caregivers. These studies are examining how computers can provide information and support through:

- *Computer-based bulletin boards*
- *Chat rooms*
- *Q&A modules*
- *Medical advice forums*

National Support for Caregivers

These computer-based support systems have become very popular because they reach many people at once, they provide privacy and convenience, and they are available around the clock.

> **Alzheimer's Association (1-800-272-3900; www.alz.org)**
> Local chapters provide referrals to area resources and services, and sponsor the **Safe Return Program**, support groups, and educational programs.

Amira C. Tame, A.C.C.

Eldercare Locator (1-800-677-1116; www.eldercare.gov)
Nationwide service of the Federal Government helps caregivers
locate local support and resources:

Alzheimer's Disease Education and Referral (ADEAR) Center
(1-800-438-4380; *www.alzheimers.org*)

**The Alzheimer's Disease Education and Referral (ADEAR)
Center** is a service of the National Institute on Aging (NIA).
The Center is a source of information and referrals for health
and social service professionals, people with Alzheimer's disease
and their families, and the general public.

- For a list of the NIA-funded Alzheimer's Disease Centers located
  throughout the U.S., contact the ADEAR Center.
- The Center produces and distributes a variety of publications
  about the disease. Information specialists are available to answer
  questions about Alzheimer's disease through a toll-free telephone
  line and through e-mail.
- The Center's Web site provides comprehensive information about
  AD. Publications can be ordered via the Web site as well.
- You can also contact the Center if you are interested in participating
  in clinical trials or donating your brain for Alzheimer's disease
  research. The NIA needs healthy people, as well as people with
  Alzheimer's disease and other dementias, to serve as volunteers.

SEE APPENDIX FOR A LIST OF
MANY MORE RESOURCES

Researchers Seek Treatments for Behavioral Symptoms

While the medical community searches for a cure for Alzheimer's disease,
there are many avenues to pursue to alleviate symptoms and suffering
for individuals and their families. The most important avenues are
family/caregiver education, support services, and activities.

Non-drug approaches include planned *therapeutic and mentally stimulating
activities* (exercise, recreation, art, music, and pet therapy). Activities are
continually being reviewed and improved by researchers, family members,

and caregivers who wish to help individuals with Alzheimer's disease enjoy the best possible quality of life. Alzheimer's causes behavioral symptoms within the brain that are not intentional or controllable by the individual. Anxiety, agitation, repetitiveness, wandering, shouting, and sleeplessness are typical symptoms. These behaviors usually appear in combination with others and make them more difficult to manage.

The Alzheimer's Association funds research on behavioral treatments to help individuals and their families cope with changes that accompany the disease. Currently, researchers are investigating a variety of behavioral treatments and strategies, including:

- Behavioral symptoms such as agitation, shouting, or sleeplessness are often a result of pain and discomfort that an individual with dementia cannot express. By being able to identify and treat pain and discomfort, health care professionals, caregivers, and family members can improve quality of life for individuals with Alzheimer's.
- Often, individuals with Alzheimer's disease become aggressive and agitated for reasons unknown to their caregivers. Researchers are identifying factors that may trigger aggressive behavior in people with Alzheimer's and developing interventions that may lessen or prevent these behaviors from occurring.
- Increasing caregiver and family involvement in their daily activities can improve the quality of life for all individuals affected by the disease.
- Providing support through family intervention can decrease depression and feelings of burden frequently experienced by caregivers, and may improve behavior, communication, and function in individuals with the disease.

Researchers are currently searching for new ways to effectively treat behavioral symptoms and improve quality of life for individuals with Alzheimer's disease and their families with non-drug therapy.

A person with Alzheimer's disease may no longer be able to do math but still be able to read magazines with pleasure for months or years to come. Playing the piano might become too stressful in the face of increasing mistakes, but singing along with others may be satisfying.

Amira C. Tame, A.C.C.

The chess board may have to be put away, but one may still be able to play tennis.

Despite the many exasperating moments, many opportunities remain for positive interactions.

The American Academy of Neurology, an association of more than 17,700 neurologists and neuroscience professionals, is dedicated to improving care through education and research.

For the study, 1,772 people age 65 or older, who were determined to be non-demented at the time of baseline assessment, were evaluated over a seven-year period. The study subjects were a representative sample of residents from three census tracts in North Manhattan, New York. Clinical data was gathered at an initial assessment, and subjects were categorized according to age, ethnicity, education level and occupation. They then reported their participation in 13 common leisure activities categorized as intellectual, physical and social pursuits.

"Even when controlling for factors like ethnic group, education and occupation, subjects with high leisure activity had 38 percent less risk of developing dementia," according to the study. The study also showed that participation in leisure activities may have a cumulative effect, with an additional 8 percent risk reduction associated with each leisure activity engaged. All three activity categories were shown to be beneficial, although the intellectual activities were associated with highest risk reduction.

For baseline clinical data, a physician elicited each subject's medical and neurological history and conducted a physical and neurological examination. All subjects also received neuropsychological testing. The evaluation was repeated at each follow-up event, and it was determined whether or not participants became demented.

Once considered a rare disorder, Alzheimer's disease is now seen as a major public health problem because of its impact on millions of older Americans and their families. As a result, research into AD has grown dramatically. Thousands of scientists in laboratories and institutions all over the world are working hard to unravel the secrets of AD and find ways to lessen its impact and perhaps, someday, to prevent it.

Treatment

Apart from treating the specific symptoms of Alzheimer' disease, it is important to observe the general state of health. A good general condition improves their feeling of well-being. An increasing degree of confusion, restlessness and aggressive behavior caused by physical illness can hinder progress with activities.

Care and the organization of the environment can ease the complication of conditions associated with Alzheimer's disease. These conditions are a concern in particular for the caregivers as well as the person suffering with this disease. Improvements can be achieved through physical, emotional and mental intervention.

There is help for many physical problems such as incontinence, difficulties of food intake, and problems with walking, sitting, lying down, etc.

In any stage, training of thinking and memory functions should be carried out carefully, otherwise there is the danger that diminishing mental abilities will be highlighted. There is no cure for Alzheimer's, but medication and *therapeutic activities* can improve the symptoms and can slow down the progression.

There are a number of drugs on the market today that can improve brain function. Typically antidementia or psychotropic drugs are prescribed. These treatments include:

- □ beta adrenergic blockers
- □ anti-seizure medications
- □ cholinesterase inhibitors
- □ antipsychotic drugs
- □ antidepressants

As AD gradually erodes memory and mental abilities, it also begins to change a person's emotions and personality. Over the course of the disease, most people (70% to 90%) eventually develop some behavioral symptoms, including sleeplessness, wandering and pacing, aggression, agitation, anger, depression, and hallucinations and delusions. These behaviors may become worse as the day comes to an end (Sundowner's Syndrome), or during daily routines such as bathing.

Most experts advise caregivers to try a variety of techniques to manage troublesome behaviors and only prescribe drugs when the behavior has become too difficult for the caregiver to handle. Symptoms are one of the hardest aspects of the disease for family and caregivers to deal with.

Researchers are slowly learning more about why they occur and are studying new treatments—drug and non-drug—to deal with them.

What are the diagnostic tests used in Alzheimer's disease?

Currently, Alzheimer's disease cannot be diagnosed with 100 percent certainty until a brain autopsy is performed upon someone's death. Non-invasive imaging procedures, such as a CAT scan or an MRI, and cognitive-behavioral tests that are easy to administer can diagnose Alzheimer's at its earliest stages or even before it starts. These tests are only part of the process, however, the diagnosis rests largely on the judgment of a physician experienced in handling dementing illnesses. Physicians may conduct a series of tests in order to rule out other possibilities.

Early Diagnosis is Important

Early diagnosis is important for the following reasons:

1) **For dementias that are reversible (an estimated 10%), more complete recovery is possible.**
2) **Morbidity of contributing conditions reduced.**
3) **Earlier interventions reduce caregiver stress and burden.**
4) **The person with Alzheimer's can be involved in decision-making.**
5) **Treatment is easier to implement and more likely to be effective.**

The Effects of Alzheimer's Disease

Damage to the brain can cause a person to act in altered or unpredictable ways. Some individuals become anxious or aggressive, while others repeat certain questions or gestures. Challenging behaviors not only cause discomfort to individuals with the disease but also can be frustrating and stressful for caregivers who cannot understand them.

Caregivers need to recognize that not all behavioral symptoms are problematic. If a certain behavior does not cause difficulties for the individual with Alzheimer's, the caregiver, or anyone else, the best strategy may be to do nothing. However, if a particular behavior becomes problematic or harmful, many health care professionals and researchers recommend methods other than drugs as the first strategy for treatment.

Changes in behavior may be prompted by several factors:

- Not able to express physical discomfort or pain they are experiencing.
- Fear of unfamiliar surroundings or loud noises that accompany active environments.
- Frustration due to their inability to communicate clearly or perform daily activities once familiar to them.

Behavioral symptoms also result from adverse reactions to common occurrences and may stem from fear and anxiety caused by memory loss, confusion and disorientation. They may be frustrated by their decreasing abilities and increasing dependence upon caregivers. Behavioral problems do not always become apparent immediately after onset of disease and often change as the disease progresses.

The outlook for older people is brighter than ever. The myth that older people always become inactive or experience great loss of mental and physical abilities is being dispelled as researchers identify some of the keys to successful aging.

At the same time, however, we are learning more about a tremendous threat to the health and well-being of all older Americans: Alzheimer's disease and other dementias.

In some respects, Alzheimer's disease is still a mystery. There is much we still don't know about why some people develop it and others don't and how to treat or prevent it. But this mystery is steadily being unraveled and our knowledge is increasing every day.

Chapter 2

Caregiver Treatment: Confront Your Anger and Frustration

Take Time

Take time to laugh
It is the music of the soul.

Take time to think
It is the source of power.

Take time to play
It is the source of perpetual youth.

Take time to read
It is the fountain of wisdom.

Take time to pray
It is the greatest power on earth.

Take time to love and be loved
It is a God-given privilege.

Take time to be friendly
It is the road to happiness.

Take time to give
It is too short a day to be selfish.

Take time to work, paid or voluntary
It is the price of success.

—Anonymous

Amira C. Tame, A.C.C.

You Are Not Alone

Each day more than 22 million Americans devote all or part of their day assisting 4 million older family members, neighbors or friends who wish to remain at home and independent of nursing homes or other long-term care facilities. Caregivers include spouses (who are often elderly themselves), as well as siblings, children, grandchildren and other family members.

Part of the difficulty among some caregivers is their many other responsibilities. Studies show 75% of caregivers are women, 25% of whom care for older parents and younger children. Over 50% of caregivers also work outside the home. Many of these caregivers find the demands of their careers and caregiving responsibilities in conflict with each other. When this happens, it is important for caregivers to discuss their needs with their employers.

In 1993, the Family and Medical Leave Act was introduced to ensure employers address the needs of their employees with regard to elder care and parenting. Emphasis is currently being placed on expanding those efforts. An increasing number of companies and government agencies at all levels are offering flex-time, job-sharing or rearranging of work schedules to help caregivers minimize their stress. Many companies also offer resource materials, counseling and training programs to assist caregivers with their responsibilities.

In addition, a formal proclamation was issued by President Clinton in 1996 designating the week of Thanksgiving as National Caregivers Week, a week set aside each year for the nation to honor and support the daily contributions of family caregivers across the United States.

Caring for someone with Alzheimer's disease is demanding and often frustrating. It is difficult to accept that your loved one, who was once full of love, energy, and inspiration, is now forgetful and totally dependent on you. In the advanced stages of the disease they will need your assistance for some of the simplest functions, such as using the restroom, putting on shoes, remembering to take medications, etc.

For many caregivers, it is perfectly normal to experience feelings of fear. You may fear that your loved one will never get better, or have a fear of not knowing what she/he will forget next.

You may fear it could be yourself that is soon forgotten. You may fear you are gradually losing someone you have been very close to. Have you recently felt trapped? Impatient? Have you begun to react to stress with your emotions and feelings instead of logic and reason? Take heart in knowing you are not alone. All of these fears are natural and predictable reactions to this devastating disease.

This book has been written with you, the caregiver, in mind. I will teach you how to develop the capacity to work with and help those afflicted with this debilitating disease. Many years of observation through group and one-on-one therapeutic activity sessions, have convinced me that you can overcome your fears and make positive differences for the person with Alzheimer's and yourself. My techniques will help through the maze of confusion and direct a path toward a quality life style.

Following these guidelines will help you to move beyond the emotional road blocks and give you a better understanding of how to cope with the many difficulties you will be facing. In addition to reducing your feelings of fear and frustration, you will feel relieved and satisfied when you see memory improvement, restored relationships, and an enhanced quality of life. Many caregivers have witnessed improvement in recipients of these therapeutic activities and techniques.

Understanding Caregiver Stress

Everyone has stress in their life every day. Stress can be created at work, trying to accomplish difficult tasks, or from expectations you put upon yourself. Stress can be dominant in the home with financial or family issues that seem insurmountable. You can have stress at play, in stop and go traffic, confronting difficult situations etc. Pressure to perform can be stressful for some and a major catastrophe for others. These everyday life stresses are usually temporary. Much of our personal stress can be reduced by rearranging our schedules, changing our expectations, avoiding stressful situations, etc.

A person suffering from Alzheimer's disease is unable to change the progression of the disease without help. You can learn how to effectively help the one who really suffers from this devastating disease. Their stress will not go away without your help. It will not go away with time. Without your help, it only gets worse.

Keep in mind that you did not cause this devastating disease, and neither did the person suffering from it. Unwarranted guilty feelings are counterproductive. The effects of Alzheimer's has caused the stress and agony you feel as a caregiver. Doing the following will help you maintain a positive attitude and disposition:

1. Make a list of the most important things in your life.
2. Define the most important goals you need to achieve and prioritize them.
3. Create a plan that has realistic goals you can achieve.
4. Keep accurate records of all positive events, actions, results, credits and achievements.
5. Remind yourself of your personal achievements and that none would have been possible without the proper knowledge and tools.

Minimize Your Negative Feelings

Caregivers often erroneously convince themselves that Alzheimer's disease is the root cause of their anxieties and there is no positive resolution available. It is essential to minimize your feelings of anger, frustration, and hopelessness so you can maximize the effectiveness of the tools and techniques described in this book. To effectively control these negative feelings, you must take appropriate steps to resolve the underlying issues.

Alzheimer's disease itself is not the root cause of a caregiver's anxiety. The anxiety comes from feeling helpless to alter or prevent the deteriorating condition of your loved one, particularly if you have a close relationship with the person you're caring for. Your relationship may need to be redefined with a new set of expectations.

Status quo is no longer an option. Without hard work and understanding on your part, the relationship can worsen and you will eventually move further apart from someone you truly care for. Although Alzheimer's disease is progressive, the *symptoms* can be minimized and the quality of life for Alzheimer sufferers and family members greatly improved. But there is little a person with Alzheimer's can do about his/her well-being *without your help*. Most importantly, you must recognize that your loved one is suffering from a disease that causes a diminished understanding of everyone around them, including you. Everything around them is becoming unfamiliar.

If you implement these methods of therapeutic activities and learn from the many examples of actual cases provided, you will improve your ability to cope with the symptoms of this devastating disease and make significant differences in your loved one's life. Remember to *always* show understanding. Treat their past with honor and respect.

Reduce Caregiver Stress

The burden a caregiver carries can be staggering. Coping becomes difficult and things can easily drift out of control. The following are warning signs of caregiving-related stress according to the Alzheimer's Disease and Related Disorders Association:

1. **Denial** about the disease and its effect on the person who's been diagnosed. *I know Mom's going to get better.*
2. **Anger** at the person with Alzheimer's or others; that no effective treatments or cures currently exist; and that people don't understand what's going on. *If he asks me that question one more time, I'll scream!*
3. **Social withdrawal** from friends and activities that once brought pleasure. *I don't care about getting together with the neighbors anymore.*
4. **Anxiety** about facing another day and what the future holds. *What happens when he needs more care than I can provide?*
5. **Depression** begins to break your spirit and affects your ability to cope. *I don't care anymore.*
6. **Exhaustion** makes it nearly impossible to complete necessary daily tasks. *I'm too tired for this.*
7. **Sleeplessness** caused by a never-ending list of concerns. *What if s/he wanders out of the house or falls and gets hurt?*
8. **Irritability** leads to moodiness and triggers negative responses and reactions. *Leave me alone!*
9. **Lack of concentration** makes it difficult to perform familiar tasks. *I was so busy, I forgot we had an appointment.*
10. **Health problems** begin to take their toll, both mentally and physically. *I can't remember the last time I felt good.*

Amira C. Tame, A.C.C.

If you are experiencing any of these stress related symptoms, the Alzheimer's Association suggests the following actions:

1. **Get a diagnosis as early as possible**
   Symptoms of Alzheimer's may appear gradually. If a person seems physically healthy, it is easy to ignore unusual behavior or attribute it to something else. See a physician when Alzheimer warning signs are present. Some dementia symptoms are treatable. Once you know what you're dealing with, you'll be able to better manage the present and plan for the future.

2. **Know what resources are available**
   For your own well-being and that of the person you are caring for, become familiar with Alzheimer care resources available in your community. Adult day care, in-home assistance, visiting nurses and Meals-on-Wheels are just a few of the community services that can offer help. Your local Alzheimer's Association chapter is also a good place to start.

3. **Become an educated caregiver**
   As Alzheimer's progresses, different caregiving skills and capabilities are necessary. Care techniques and suggestions available from the Alzheimer's Association can help you better understand and cope with many of the challenging behaviors and personality changes.

4. **Get help**
   Trying to do everything yourself will leave you exhausted. Support of family, friends and community resources can be an enormous help. If assistance is not offered, ask for it. And if you have difficulty asking for assistance, have someone close to you do it. If stress becomes overwhelming, don't be afraid to seek professional help. Alzheimer's Association support groups and helplines are also good sources of comfort and reassurance.

5. **Take care of yourself**
   Caregivers frequently devote themselves totally to those they care for, and in the process, neglect their own needs. Pay attention to yourself. Watch your diet, exercise and get plenty of rest. Use respite services to take time off for shopping, a movie or an uninterrupted

visit with a friend. Those close to you, including your loved one who has Alzheimer's, want you to take care of yourself.

6. **Manage your level of stress**
Stress can cause physical problems (blurred vision, stomach irritation, high blood pressure) and changes in behavior (irritability, lack of concentration, loss of appetite). Note your symptoms. Use relaxation techniques that work for you and consult a physician if necessary.

7. **Accept changes as they occur**
People with Alzheimer's change, and so do their needs. Eventually they may require care beyond what you can provide at home. A thorough investigation of available care options should make transitions easier, as will support and assistance from those who care about you and your loved one.

8. **Do legal and financial planning**
Consult an attorney and discuss issues related to durable power of attorney, living wills and trusts, future medical care, housing and other key considerations. Planning now will alleviate stress later. If possible, involve your loved one and other family members in planning activities and decisions.

9. **Be realistic**
Until a cure is found, the progression of Alzheimer's disease is inevitable. The care you provide does make a difference. Neither you nor the person with Alzheimer's can control many of the circumstances and behaviors that will occur. Give yourself permission to grieve for the losses you experience, but also focus on the positive moments as they occur and enjoy your good memories.

10. **Give yourself credit, not guilt**
You're only human. Occasionally, you lose patience and are unable to provide all the care you would like. But you are doing the best you can, so give yourself credit. Being a devoted caregiver is not something to feel guilty about. Your loved one needs you and you are there, so be proud. And if your loved one could thank you, they would.

Once you discover there is still quality time you can spend with your loved one, you will want to get close again to him/her. As you witness positive changes in attitude and memory functions, you will become more confident utilizing the techniques discussed in this book. It is important to understand you can help yourself *and* your loved one *and* enjoy doing it. Knowing you truly have a positive impact on someone suffering from dementia is a powerful healer of caregiver stress.

Reducing the intensity of negative emotional feelings the person with Alzheimer's is feeling can sometimes help improve a caregiver's outlook. As we realize the positive effects of therapeutic activities, our own frustrations turn into relief and satisfaction because we have made a positive difference in someone's life.

As you complete the Personal Profile Form in Chapter 3, you will be asked information about your loved one's past that will be helpful during the activities treatment program. Gathering pictures to stimulate positive thoughts with your loved one will also help you recall the good times from the past. Writing down what your loved one liked and disliked in the past will help to recall who he really was and how much he/she means to you. Once you complete the survey, you will have made the first step toward renewing your lost relationship.

Care for the Caregiver

Your thoughts may be centered around the person in your household who currently needs the most nursing and nurturing—your loved one with Alzheimer's or other dementia disorders, but it is important to remember that as a caregiver, you need tender loving care too!

The following are self-help strategies for caregivers:

Take time off for yourself. Plan time away from the task of 24-hour care. Do something just for you! There are qualified professionals available who can give you a break and also provide a change.

Take time off with the whole family. Do something suitable for everyone, but make it a special occasion, whether it is a picnic or a trip to wherever you wish. If your loved one is unable to attend, take photos or a video to share when you return.

Meet and talk with others. There is benefit from talking with other people who are familiar with what you are going through. Commiserating, venting, and laughing together can go a long way toward relieving your burden. Try meeting in a mutual support chat online or on a message board, or find a local "offline" support group. Your family member's or friend's primary health care provider may refer you to a local support network. Explore and use the resources of the many nationwide and community-oriented volunteer organizations, including the local chapter of the Alzheimer's Association.

Avoid isolation, as it can lead to depression. Invite a neighbor or friend to join a club with you. This may be the time to begin an exercise or walking program for your health. Start a hobby you've always been interested in that includes others, e.g., line dancing, golf, bowling. Don't say there is no time. This is your prescription for good health!

Get extra help! This could include help for chores around the house or a professional activities therapist. Contact the Alzheimer's Association in your area to steer you in the right direction.

Visit your loved one's health care provider. Be assertive in getting the information you feel you need. Take along a list of questions to ask the clinician. Don't leave until you have received answers you feel comfortable with. Alzheimer's disease affects the ability to express what is hurting or to describe other health issues.

Caregivers' Rights

As you take on the challenge of caring for the person suffering from Alzheimer's disease, more and more of your freedom and self-identity are absorbed by your new role as caregiver. Therefore, you must remind yourself of your rights as a human being and a loving caregiver. Some of the rights that are easy to lose focus of are:

- To be treated with respect.
- To not have all the answers.
- To seek help from others.

- To experience stress, anger and lack of control without guilt.
- To occasional freedom from the duty of caregiving.
- To feel overwhelmed with the responsibility of caring for your loved one.
- To place your loved one in an Alzheimer's care facility without feeling guilty.

Chapter 3

Gathering and Discovering
Important Information

Now that you . . .

understand the effects of Alzheimer's disease and how caregivers can reduce feelings of anger, frustration, and helplessness,

You are ready to . . .

. . . learn as much as you can about the person with Alzheimer's, including historical and current data.

Amira C. Tame, A.C.C.

Why Should Information Be Gathered?

The first step in any problem-solving methodology is to gather all of the information associated with the problem. Without pertinent information surrounding the situation, your only recourse is trial and error. For people suffering from Alzheimer's disease, too many errors could do irreparable harm to the person you are caring for and the relationship you are trying to build.

You will use the information gathered in this chapter to design activities that work toward advancing your goals outlined in Chapter 4. You will also use this chapter as a reference throughout the activities program to maximize the effectiveness of each activity and speed the recovery process. The likelihood that you will see improvement in the person you are caring for without using information gathered in this chapter is very slim. You wouldn't consider preparing a meal for the first time without knowing what the ingredients are, the most effective way to combine them, how long they should cook and at what temperatures, etc. Without a recipe or someone showing you how, you wouldn't know where to begin. Eventually, through trial and error, you may produce a resemblance to the intended meal, but chances are, you threw out many botched meals. The same is true when caring for a person with Alzheimer's; however, you don't have the luxury of time or expendable resources to waste. Each success is a stepping stone to the next success until you've laid a foundation to build self-confidence and self-esteem.

If you were an employer interviewing someone for a particular job, you would certainly want to know some history of the person's experience and performance. You would want to ensure that the applicant's skills and abilities matched the requirements for the position being offered. A mismatch would only cause fear, anxiety, confusion, anger, etc. Sound familiar? You don't want the person you are caring for to be subjected to similar mismatched expectations. Just as a resumé provides pertinent information for the employer to direct questions to the candidate and assess abilities, the Personal Profile Form will give you historical data and personality traits needed to match activities to goals and abilities.

You will also gather information about likes and dislikes to improve the success rate of your activities. Suggesting activities the person enjoys will encourage participation and lead to a closer relationship. They will see you as someone who likes the same things he/she does. Even if you are a caregiver who is a close relative or someone who has cared for this person a long time, it's important to complete the survey questions to help you ease the burden and bring back some of the good memories as you gather the information.

Learning about close and trusted family members and close friends will give you insight into what type of personalities they chose to be close to. Knowing the person's personality will help in establishing a good relationship.

Work and educational history can provide significant background information they may be very willing to talk about. Medical information, including any information about long-term illness, and medication or limitations associated with medical or physical conditions are necessary for you to respond to specific needs.

Why This Information Is So Important

Understanding the person with Alzheimer's will considerably improve your communication as you are designing and implementing a successful activity program.

Knowing the person you are caring for will alleviate much of the stress associated with trial and error. Alzheimer's care is a very challenging task. You owe it to yourself and the person you're caring for to do everything possible to minimize mistakes that are counterproductive toward achieving your goals.
Get to know as much as possible to help you understand what personality traits and memory functions have been affected by Alzheimer's disease. Anything that has changed as a result of this disease is an area of potential improvement.

A person with a strong personality (bossy) will probably continue to be strong-minded even with Alzheimer's disease. It is unlikely that you will be able to change behavior or a personality that was a lifelong trait. Sometimes a personality trait will become even stronger as fear of losing one's identity sets in.

What Information Do You Need?

Is anyone in the household allergic to cats, grass, flowers, etc.? Do they enjoy flowers (some don't)? If so, which are their favorite flowers? Are there favorite colors? Was the person physically active in earlier years? A sports lover? An active walker? A jogger? Can they eat alone? Can s/he dress without assistance? Did s/he have a serious or good-natured personality as a younger person? These are just a few of the questions that you need to answer to be able to properly design an activities program.

1. *Personality*—Understanding the person's personality will help you optimize communication by designing corresponding activities. There are three distinct personality types:

    a. Visual—Responds to pictures or written requests. Enjoys quietly watching TV. etc.
    b. Auditory—Vocalizes most thoughts freely. Responds to questions with long dissertations.
    c. Kinesthetic—Expresses emotions and likes to touch and feel items. Easily recognizes things by holding or touching them.

    Determine which of these personality types best describe the person you are working with and note this information in the Personal Profile Form in this chapter. Next, try to determine other personality traits. Were they easygoing, funny, serious, a people lover, a loner, stubborn, aggressive, critical, dominating, etc.? This information should also be recorded.

2. *Previous careers or positions*—Typically, individuals with Alzheimer's recall the earlier periods of their lives. These periods are usually full of fond memories of childhood, exciting memories of their teenage years, and favorite memories of their early working years. These periods are full of youth, adventure, and accomplishments.

    It is very important that the caregiver determine which part of the person's life can be recalled best and focus on drawing out positive memories whenever possible. It is so important for them to understand they can still remember some things whether positive or negative.

This will reduce the fear and anxiety of losing their memory and quite possibly enhance their ability to communicate and be understood.

As a caregiver, it is very important you understand that we are all unique individuals with life experiences that have shaped our past. We all have different lives and backgrounds. As we live our lives, we experience significant events that take place at various periods in our lives, and emotionally we have our highs and lows during those stages. Consider the intensity of emotions and involvement necessary to rear children until they leave home, and the experiences etched in your memory. Consider the memories of work experiences gathered through possibly two thirds of your life. As you become a little older, your life usually calms down somewhat. It makes sense that most people would recall their child-rearing years most vividly because so much time, effort, and repetition was spent during those years.

They are simply recalling events that are etched most vividly in their long term memory. Other events that seem to remain in their memory include World War II, the Great Depression, and an interest in sports, to name a few.

Once you understand the period(s) that they can best recall, you can prepare appropriate activities accordingly. You'll know from which era to select music, fashion, and determine which world events they would likely remember.

Designing activities that evolve around and are based upon what they did during their past careers is always effective and rewarding. For a person who worked in the medical field, activities involving medical events, clothing, and other related items seem to be of most interest. Those who were carpenters enjoy carpentry activities and conversation about their trade the most.

3. *Hobbies*—the things they liked to do and used to get pleasure and satisfaction out of, such as sports (football, basketball, . . .), games, crafts, etc. They may have played or participated in the hobby/activity or just enjoyed watching. Knowing whether they were active or passive participants will help you direct the level of their involvement.

4. ***Medical History & Current Health Conditions***—knowing all the medical problems, allergies, and limitations is clearly very essential in order to design your activities.

5. ***Significant Events***—such as graduations, landing first job, buying first car or television, marriage, wars, death of a president, home/favorite sport team winning the series, etc. Be careful not to dwell on negative events. Try to avoid subjects that are sad and may put them in a bad mood.

6. ***Likes and Dislikes***—

    a. ***Food/Drinks***—They may not remember favorite foods or how to prepare them. It might be very stimulating for them to enjoy food they once liked. Helping prepare a favorite dish could bring back fond memories.
    b. ***Entertainment***—This is another area with an abundance of information, such as music, movies, or sports, to use in building your activities program.
    c. ***Clothes, Colors, Smells***, etc.

How and Where Do You Obtain the Information?

1. *Family members, friends and other people who had close contact with them*—The most knowledgeable sources are immediate family such as the wife, husband, siblings, parents. The second source of information would be close friends, associates, and colleagues. The third is professionals like their doctors, lawyers, accountants, etc.

2. *Personal items and belongings*—such as photo albums can provide you with a wealth of information about family members, friends, jobs, hobbies, habits, likes, etc. A personal cook book with marked up favorite recipes can be an excellent source of favorite foods and recipes to use as activities.

3. *The person with Alzheimer's—Direct Questions*—In early stages of Alzheimer's disease they often remember valuable information they are willing to share. Sometimes they will remember something

significant about a past experience, but not many details. This may give you enough information to work with.

Effective techniques can be simple and subtle, for example, looking through photo albums. Ask questions about the pictures. Allow him/her to respond openly, and carefully listen for the information you need.

4. *Indirect—By observation*. Although the initial survey form is invaluable, you probably will not be able to fill in every blank before beginning your activity program. More information will be discovered about each individual during one-on-one sessions. That is why your observations as a caregiver are very important in learning valuable facts about the person you're caring for.

    Study their body language and eye contact to determine likes and dislikes. As you progress with activity therapy, there will be many opportunities to update the survey form.

    Show dated objects, such as a popular car models from their era, popular songs, movies, significant events, popular personalities/stars, wars, and disasters. Observe and listen to their remarks and reactions. Reviewing dated activities and events will help you determine the time periods they still recall.

The following forms will assist you in recording and organizing the pertinent information utilized throughout your activities program.

Amira C. Tame, A.C.C.

Personal Profile Form

Personal Data

Name of Client _____

SSN _____ Case No. _____

Date of intake into facility or date activities sessions began _____

Age: _____ Gender: ☐ Male   ☐ Female

Place of birth _____ ☐ City   ☐ Rural   ☐ Farm

How long at present address? _____

Religion (optional) _____

Languages spoken (other than English) _____

Name of primary contact _____

Relationship _____

Phone: Office _____ Home _____

Emergency Contact:

Name _____ Relationship _____

Phone: Office _____ Home _____

Name _____ Relationship _____

Phone: Office _____ Home _____

Home/Resident Care Facility _____

Address _____

Phone _____ Administrator _____

Primary Physician _____ Phone _____

Medical Specialist _____ Phone _____

Immediate family members and close friends:

Name	Relation	Telephone
_____	_____	_____
_____	_____	_____
_____	_____	_____
_____	_____	_____
_____	_____	_____

Where did he/she spend most of his/her childhood? Type of area:
☐ Rural   ☐ Farm   ☐ City   ☐ Other

High School (Prom, graduation, girl friends, jobs, education, etc.)

_____

_____

_____

_____

Medical Conditions (high blood pressure, diabetes, high/low sugar, arthritis, sensitive skin [bruise easily], react to chemicals, etc.)

_____

_____

_____

_____

Physical Limitations (blindness, hearing loss, restricted movement, etc.)

_____

_____

_____

_____

History of Mental Illness

_____

_____

_____

_____

Allergies (allergic to chemicals, bee stings, medications or over-the-counter drugs, flowers, grass, etc.)

_____

_____

_____

_____

Adaptive Aids Used/Needed
☐ Hearing Aid   ☐ Prosthetic devises   ☐ Dentures
☐ Clothing   ☐ Special eating equipment   ☐ Glasses

☐ Wheelchair   ☐ Ambulatory equipment
☐ Walkers   ☐ Breathing apparatus
☐ Others

_____ _____

_____ _____

_____ _____

Info. Received From _____ **Date** _____
Care facility, primary caregiver, physician

Medication	*Prescribed by*
1. _____	_____
2. _____	_____
4. _____	_____
5. _____	_____
6. _____	_____

Doctor's Name	*Telephone #*	*Specialty*
1. _____	_____	_____
2. _____	_____	_____
3. _____	_____	_____
4. _____	_____	_____
5. _____	_____	_____

Unusual/Uncommon Behaviors (a twitch, limp, stutter, involuntary movements, etc.)

1. _____

_____

2. _____

_____

3. _____

_____

4. _____

_____

5. _____

_____

6. _____

_____

Things that may be agitating
1. _____
   _____
2. _____
   _____
3. _____
   _____
4. _____
   _____
5. _____
   _____
6. _____
   _____

Things that might be calming

1. Special phrases or subjects _____
   _____
   _____
   _____

2. Certain food, drink, dessert items _____
   _____
   _____
   _____

3. Activities (radio, television, etc.)_____
   _____
   _____
   _____

4. Calming medications_____
   _____
   _____
   _____

5. Other _____
   _____
   _____
   _____

Amira C. Tame, A.C.C.

Personality

Personality type (see page 5)   □ Visual   □ Auditory   □ Kinesthetic

_____

_____

Personality traits (funny, serious, spontaneous, generous, loner, critical, dominating, content, aggressive, neat, organized, moody, antisocial, etc.)

Before Alzheimer's disease   **Current traits**

_____   _____

_____   _____

_____   _____

_____   _____

                                           _____

                                           _____

Personality disorders (if any) _____

_____

_____

_____

Career
Did they have a professional career history
(inside or outside the home)? _____ How many years?_____
Describe the history of the career _____

_____

_____

Explain in detail the responsibilities, skills, achievements, etc.
Primary Job: _____ How Long?_____
Description_____

_____

_____

Secondary Job: _____ How Long?_____
Description _____
_____
_____

Secondary Job: _____ How Long?_____
Description _____
_____
_____

List the type of tools and equipment used (hammer, bulldozer, car, truck, computer, telephone, etc.)

1. _____   5. _____
2. _____   6. _____
3. _____   7. _____
4. _____   8. _____

Distinctive clothes or uniforms they wore:

1. _____   3. _____
2. _____   4. _____

Food

Did he/she enjoy cooking at home, eating out, or a combination of both?

_____
_____
_____

What types of food did he/she enjoy (ethnic, Italian, American, Chinese, Middle Eastern, etc.)? _____

_____
_____

List foods they enjoyed in the following categories starting with the most favorite:

	1st Choice	2nd Choice	3rd Choice	4th Choice
Meats	_____	_____	_____	_____
Vegetables	_____	_____	_____	_____
Dairy Prod.	_____	_____	_____	_____

Fruits   _____   _____   _____   _____
Breads   _____   _____   _____   _____
Cereals   _____   _____   _____   _____
Pastas   _____   _____   _____   _____
Desserts   _____   _____   _____   _____
Spices   _____   _____   _____   _____
Snacks   _____   _____   _____   _____
Beverages   _____   _____   _____   _____

List foods favored during the following meal times:
Breakfast   _____   _____   _____   _____
Lunch   _____   _____   _____   _____
Dinner   _____   _____   _____   _____

Entertainment
Favorite form of entertainment ? _____
_____
_____

Favorite movies (funny, action, drama, musical, political) _____
_____
_____

Favorite actors/actresses _____
_____

Favorite music (classical, opera, Motown, jazz, blues, country, big band)
_____
_____

Favorite singers _____
_____
_____

Favorite songs _____
_____
_____

Musical instrument(s) played (if any), and at what level (beginner, professional, etc.)
_____
_____

Sports (football, basketball, baseball, hockey, etc.—note whether they were an active participant or a spectator) _____

_____

_____

Did the individual enjoy playing games (cards, word games, board games, active games like charades, etc.)? _____

_____

_____

Hobbies, Games, Puzzles

List the individual's hobbies (may include gardening, sports, watching TV, listening to music, reading, painting, writing, bird watching, woodworking, playing card games, board games, Dominoes, Bingo, crafts, knitting, sewing, stamp/doll/car/coin collecting, basket weaving, puzzles, model building). Be specific. Was s/he an active (A) participant or a spectator (S)?

1. _____
2. _____
3. _____
4. _____
5. _____

Clothing
What kind of clothes s/he liked to wear. What materials s/he liked and felt comfortable in. _____

_____

_____

Colors liked/disliked _____

_____

_____

_____

Did s/he enjoy shopping for clothes? ☐ No ☐ Yes
If yes, where/style, etc. _____
Did s/he enjoy visiting the mall? ☐ No ☐ Yes
If yes, what stores _____

Does the individual enjoy a wide variety of clothes? ☐ No ☐ Yes
If yes, what styles _____

Scheduled Daily Events

(to help coordinate activities sessions)

List their daily routine events. This includes TV shows, walks, doctor visits, meals, snack time, naps, scheduled visits, group activities (clubs, church, sporting events, etc.)

	Event	Day(s)	Time
1.			
2.			
3.			
4.			
5.			
6.			
7.			
8.			
9.			
10.			
11.			
12.			
13.			
14.			
15.			
16.			
17.			
18.			

Intake Goals—Assessment

Intake Date _____ Client Name _____ Assessment Date _____

Goals	Priority	None	Some	Moderate	Significant
How Am I Doing? Improvements					
The following goals target essential changes that will improve the quality of life for people suffering from Alzheimer's disease. You may be experiencing some or all of the underlying symptoms at some level. Some symptoms may be subtle and others may be dramatic. To help you plan and monitor an appropriate activity program, please check the goal box that describes the changes you would like to make, prioritize them, and evaluate improvement levels.					
Repair damaged or lost relationships					
Reduce negative emotions,e.g., fear, anger, frustration, guilt					
Change antisocial behavior, e.g. participating in group activities					
Improve physical appearance, e.g., haircuts, makeup, general grooming					
Willingness to use good hygiene, e.g., bathing, brushing teeth					
Improve memory function—recall past / learn new things					
Understand and accept the disease and give hope for improving my quality of life					
Reduce wandering and confusion about living arrangements					
Improve self-confidence					
Improve eating habits					
Utilize physical motor skills to improve strength and coordination					
Reduce violent behavior					
Increase mobility					
Reduce mood swings					
Other					
Comments:					

Amira C. Tame, A.C.C.

Activities Progress Report

Client: _____ Case No.: _____

Therapist: _____

Date: _____ Date of Previous Session: _____

Attitude

(Responsiveness and Willingness to Participate)

Today's Session
____ Excellent
____ Good
____ Fair
____ Poor

Since Previous Session
____ Improved
____ Same
____ Slight Improvement
____ Worse

Responsiveness to Activities

Activity	Very	Somewhat	None	Comments
Music				
Art				
Craft				
Games				
Flower Arranging				
Exercise				
Conversation				
Outing				
Walking				
Cooking				
Note any progress or deterioration of motor, auditory, sensory skills; moods, etc.				

NOTES

Amira C. Tame, A.C.C.

Chapter 4

Understanding the Concepts, Tools and Techniques

Hugging

Hugging is healthy
> It helps our body's immune system, it
> keeps us healthier, it cures depression, it
> reduces stress, it induces sleep, it's
> invigorating, it's rejuvenating, it has no
> unpleasant side effects, and hugging is
> nothing less than a miracle drug.

Hugging is all natural
> It is organic, naturally sweet, no
> pesticides, no preservatives, no artificial
> ingredients and 100 percent wholesome.

Hugging is practically perfect
> There are no movable parts, no batteries
> to wear out, no periodic checkups, low
> energy consumption, high energy yield,
> inflation-proof, nonfattening, no monthly
> payments, no insurance requirements,
> theftproof, nontaxable, nonpolluting and,
> of course, fully returnable.

Amira C. Tame, A.C.C.

You Can Make a Difference

Caring for a person with Alzheimer's can be very frustrating. What works for one person may not work for another. What works to relieve symptoms one day doesn't work the next. Through many years of working with hundreds of persons with Alzheimer's, I've developed techniques and created activities that address these difficulties. The success I've experienced, using these techniques, has given me encouragement to share them with others.

Positive results are not achieved easily or quickly. Working with Alzheimer's is hard work and requires a great deal of perseverance and patience. At times, even your most sincere attempts to be helpful or to communicate are met with angry outbursts, resistance, or sometimes, complete withdrawal.

Persons with Alzheimer's often develop negative feelings such as mistrust, fear, anxiety, low self-esteem, resentment and confusion. They feel there is little or no hope for their decline in memory function. These feelings can be attributed to their diminishing ability to remember and process simple information such as dates, family member names, how to tie shoelaces, or how to use the restroom independently. As the disease progresses, confidence in their ability to accomplish *anything* makes it more difficult to get positive responses.

However, utilizing the techniques described in this chapter will help restore positive feelings and lift them from their deepest withdrawals. Furthermore, with time, each will begin to participate in and enjoy activities at their individual level of comprehension and ability. Many continue to learn new tasks and improve their memory.

I visited a resident after I had not seen her for more than a year. When she saw me and heard my voice and my laugh she looked surprised and delighted and said, "Where have you been? I missed you!" She remembered my voice and also recalled many of the activities we enjoyed together. I am convinced that some improvement is possible at almost any stage of Alzheimer's disease.

As you utilize the techniques described herein, you will see their memory function improve. You will see a dramatic improvement in some and a reduction of the symptoms in others.

Alzheimer's causes difficulties in many areas that can benefit from therapeutic activities. Listed below are areas that most issues are associated with. A form is provided in Chapter 3 to help break down main categories into more details. (Intake Goals—Assessment).

- Improve relationships.
- Reduce negative emotions, for example, fear, anger, frustration, guilt.
- Cope with and decrease unpredictable mood swings.
- Increase positive attitude and self-confidence levels.
- Develop happiness, enjoyment and self-worth.
- Improve long—and short-term memory functions.

Improve Relationships

As the relationships improve, so do communication and expression of feelings that provide important feedback to the caregiver. Positive relationships are also built upon respect, trust and self-worth.

As the disease progresses, most begin to mistrust everyone around them, including themselves, their loved ones, and caregivers. This is due to memory deterioration and inability to perform basic functions such as brushing teeth or tying shoes, uncertainty of present circumstances or of what is happening to and around them (death of a family member, what the future holds, the possibility of further deterioration from the disease, life expectancy, caregiver status).

Another reason for mistrust may be that they don't know the status of their finances or home. They often forget important details, and the one thought they continue to remember is being unsure of what's happening in their life! Be consistent when reassuring them about personal finances. Hopefully, finances are managed by an individual whom they trust. Sometimes a trip to the bank will provide assurance that accounts are in a safe place. Carrying a small amount of money with them provides a sense of financial security and independence. The person you're caring for will feel more at ease sharing thoughts and feelings if you are perceived as being trustworthy.

They may ask you not to share any of these conversations with others. Assure them that conversations between the two of you will be confidential. Without this trust, they may not want to share with you, and your ability to build a relationship will suffer.

Although trust begins with effective communication, maintaining it is a continual process. Without trust, relationships cannot be developed or maintained. Individuals with Alzheimer's are usually suspicious of everything and everyone because they are no longer sure of themselves or others.

Techniques to Help Them Reconnect

Improving relationships with family members, including caregivers and friends, provides peace of mind and reduces frustrations. Creating a loving and caring atmosphere has a positive effect on their well-being. Building activities around occasions or people who matter (especially children) are important and will lift their spirits and provide a reason to smile. Several techniques and activities to utilize include:

- Use activities that reflect good times spent with the family, such as watching video tapes or looking at photographs of joyful events (weddings/graduations of close family members and friends, births of children and grandchildren, vacations). Another activity is to create a homemade family tree poster using pictures of favorite people (include friends, pets, family).
- Find opportunities to patch sour relationships with family and old friends who haven't been seen for a while, and if possible, bring these people back into the person's life for a visit. They can probably add enjoyment, happiness and meaning to the person's life. Make sure there is willingness on both sides to reconcile the relationship. Don't force the issue, but emphasize the benefits for everyone.
- Videos and photographs are effective ways to reconnect happy occasions and important people and are constant reminders of having a loving family. An effective approach is to talk about the person on the video and say their names as you see them.
  Encourage participants to talk about their relationship and love for the person with Alzheimer's. Videotape family members

and friends while they are visiting so you can replay the video for them as an activity. Videotape familiar objects—trees, swing set, wood project, etc., if possible. If it is not possible to make a special tape, ask family members if they have a video available.
- Place pictures and mementos in the person's home to serve as reminders of past accomplishments (education, credentials, plaques, certificates, offices held, career achievements, other ceremonies, handmade arts and crafts).

Reduce Negative Emotions, i.e., Fear, Anger, Frustration and Guilt

Negative emotions are common with persons suffering from Alzheimer's and for the caregiver trying to cope with the difficulties. Because negative emotions are roadblocks, it is difficult to establish and maintain positive and constructive communication. However, with persistence and time, as roadblocks are removed they will become more receptive to communication. Techniques for reducing negative emotions should include, but not be limited to, the following:

- Suggest activities in a manner that will give options and a sense of involvement in the decision-making process.
- Play calming music or sing/hum familiar tunes.
- Stimulate conversation about familiar subjects.
- Offer ice cream, gum, or go for social outings and/or walks.
- Share old magazines, pictures or items.
- Note which activities were most effective and enjoyable.
- Learn to respond to the their actions spontaneously.

If you notice negative responses to your suggestions, change the subject to something more relaxing, e.g. going out for ice cream, taking a walk, listening to favorite music. It is important to be flexible and not insist they participate in anything unacceptable. Use your best judgment as to what they like based on your experience and the Personal Profile Form. Suggest activities that are fun and easy. If you find something they enjoy, follow up with similar activities to maintain their attention.Always show interest in an activity that works. If you participate in the game or activity, maintain a humble attitude to avoid intimidating or humiliating anyone.

For example, let them show you how to play a game even if you already know how.

Individuals with Alzheimer's want to be treated as a friend with a "glad to see you" attitude and not like sick people. If you are not a family member, let them see you as a friend or a friend of the family. Encourage them to share stories or personal anecdotes. Help them understand there are ways to help cope with this disease. Give hope rather than let them be frustrated about what they've lost or can no longer do. This is difficult for a family member caring for a loved one to do, because this person remembers their life before the disease.

At times it may be helpful to play calming music or sing to help them relax. Determine the type of music they like (either through the interview process, conversations, or experimentation). It is likely they will respond to love songs or show tunes from the past. Older songs with simple lyrics and a relaxing melody can stimulate fond memories of loved ones and past events. Many like to talk about things they did, places visited, vehicles owned, and clothes worn during the time period when a particular song was popular.

When a person talks about the past, show sincere interest. Even if you were not living in or were too young to remember the particular era, you can still enjoy learning about those days. Showing interest in their recollections helps establish and maintain a positive relationship. They appreciate it when a caregiver cares enough to listen. Show respect by listening to past accomplishments, including professional careers, high school or college years, and raising a family. Tell them how important those past accomplishments are and how important it is to talk about those accomplishments.

Sometimes they do not want to listen to music or are uninterested in looking at pictures in old magazines. Suggest a walk. This might be a walk down the hallway or to other rooms. If you are at a care facility, suggest walking together to the cafeteria to purchase a snack or drink. If possible, go for a walk or to the shopping mall.

Not all activities need to be games, puzzles or questions. They could be simply relating to the person, sharing an experience, or addressing personal issues. For example, chewing gum can be relaxing and calming, but before offering, make sure there are no problems with dentures, chewing or swallowing. Gum should always be nonstick and sugar-free.

Sometimes even the most inviting opportunities to participate in an activity do not interest the person you're caring for, especially if they have developed antisocial behavior. Allow them to participate at what you understand is their level of competence. This means you must be willing to modify your expectations and activities to match their ability.

If appropriate, try a quiet atmosphere with pleasant, soft music. Provide space while watching their behavior without intervening. If a person becomes violent—swearing, throwing things, screaming—remain calm and do not panic or express fear. Moving to a different location or room may help. Maintain a positive attitude and show you are listening. Apologize if one feels agitated by you in any way. They feel better when their feelings are acknowledged. Offer snacks, stuffed animals, or whatever evokes positive responses. Always make your suggestions in a nonthreatening way, and make it clear that it is their decision to make a change.

A person with Alzheimer's is more confident doing enjoyable and familiar things. It is important to determine which are the favorite activities, conversation subjects, places to visit, and favorite snacks or foods. If any appear anxious and nervous, simply draw on one of these favorites to help distract them from the source of anxiety and discomfort. These are described as rescue activities.

Often, just asking the person to help you with an activity will generate interest (and may help you determine areas of interest). For example, ask for help preparing a salad because you are running late. Ask if they would be willing to help by cutting lettuce, tomatoes or other vegetables. More than likely they will want to help.

An activity as simple as working with tangled string or cord can be satisfying and provide a feeling of usefulness. Ask for help because you are having difficulty with it.

This is an excellent finger, hand, and mind exercise. If the person is unwilling, use passive activities such as music or reading to stimulate a response. Ask if they would like you to read or sing. Start humming softly to see if they join you. Don't insist, but ask politely to determine interest. If they can do the activities simultaneously, it could be a transition from one activity to another.

When you are finished for the day, leave them with happy and positive thoughts. When they see you the next time, they may recall happy feelings and have a brighter outlook. Leave them with a smile whenever you can.

Cope With (and Decrease) Unpredictable Mood Swings

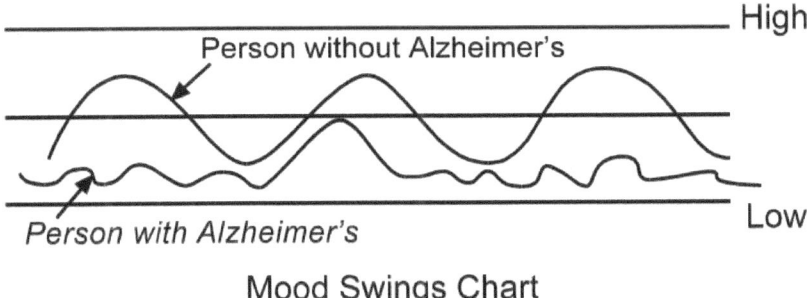

Mood Swings Chart

Mood swings are normal mood variations everyone experiences. With Alzheimer's, however, the mood swings are usually more frequent and at lower levels of happiness. Some will stay in a depressed state for an extended period of time, sometimes consciously as a result of resistant behavior or as a negative response to something said or done. Some have been in a depressed state for so long that they may fear coming out of the depression and coping with reality. They may have regressed deeply into isolation.

To be truly helpful, the caregiver must have an awareness of the person's mood swings and should try to accomplish as much as possible during an upswing period. Always be realistic and don't expect significant progress during the low emotional tides. Furthermore, keep the following points in mind:

1. Don't expect to permanently eliminate mood swings.
2. Focus on improving mood swings through empathic listening and slowly introducing appropriate activities.

3. Respect their right to have mood swings (bad days) and express an understanding of their feelings.
4. Allow quiet time without external pressure from anyone, including yourself.
5. Ask for permission to do something while you visit.

Increase Positive Attitudes and Self-Confidence

Because you can never predict a reaction, always expect the unexpected. You may find it necessary to respond with spontaneous gestures to keep their interest. Use quick, positive responses, but be certain not to hurt feelings or cause anger and dissatisfaction (and probably jeopardize your relationship). Maintaining trust and a positive relationship is a challenge you will continually need to be conscious of.

If a caregiver repeatedly responds negatively, they will, without a doubt, become angry and frustrated and begin to withdraw. Though we do not intentionally hurt the person's feelings, sometimes we misunderstand the real needs and do not respond appropriately. Thus it is essential to maintain a calming and positive atmosphere, keep communication channels open, and encourage upbeat feelings for as long as possible.

Techniques to increase positive attitudes and self-confidence include:

1. **Conversation Stimulation**
   Always begin your activity sessions with conversation. Asking general, non-invasive questions about their day is a good start. Your ability to communicate well at the beginning of a session will set the mood for the rest of your time together. Be upbeat and positive. If they are not responding, talk about your day or share an interesting story or experience. During the conversation, determine what type of activity may be appropriate to begin with. For example, if she has been in the room all day, suggest a walk either indoors or outdoors. Try to assess body language and mood to guide you in the selection of an acceptable and helpful activity.

   Passive Engagement—If the person is unresponsive to conversational or physical stimulation, then try passive activities.

Engage in an activity you are certain generated interest during past sessions. It could be something as simple as rubbing hand cream on your hands. After watching you, s/he may respond by saying that it smells good, or agree to a hand rub if you ask them.

Suggestive Encouragement—Positive feedback and constant encouragement are essential to ensure a successful activity program. There should be no serious consequences to failure. Once you have reduced their fear of failure and encouraged free and comfortable participation, you are on your way to rewarding and positive results.

Offer praise for everything said and done, even if they were simply willing to attempt the activity. Participation alone is worth recognition. Continued encouragement and praise leads to a willingness to keep trying, even though the activity may not have been successful initially.

2. **Use Familiar Activities**

Start by using activities that are easily understood to ensure success and develop a sense of accomplishment. They could be new and simple things you have been using during previous meetings.

When introducing new activities, use familiar items. If possible, use the same items in different activities. Items could be used in a seek and find game, then in a treasure hunt game. Even though the games may be different, the items are familiar. This makes it easier to be involved in the next activity. Suggested items include rings, a watch, earrings, or a favorite piece of cloth used to tie bows, make ribbons or perform simple sewing.

Choosing activities that they can be successful with involves more than using familiar items. Activities can easily be adjusted to individual levels. If success is not achieved in one level, don't abandon the activity. Modify it to fit their ability. Activities can be built upon as abilities improve. Familiar items can be added or the complexity can be increased to expand abilities as you continue with the activity. Most resistant persons will loosen up and try an activity after watching you do it. After watching you enough times, they may gain enough confidence to try the activity with you and eventually independently.

3. **Choose Activities to Fit Abilities**

Initially, choose activities they are mentally and physically capable of performing without much effort or strain. Always be sensitive and conscious of cues and subtle communications. Provide enough space for them to be spontaneous and not worry about being wrong. Patience is very important at this stage, as progress can be slow and frustrating.

Incremental Stimulation

To achieve the best results, incrementally increase the complexity of activities as abilities improve. This requires close attention by the caregiver to detect improvement in ability. Don't expect a person to be excited, behave the way you wish, follow your directions, or immediately participate in activities. You need to slowly and consciously move present levels of participation to more complicated and involved activities.

Remember, your goal is to steadily gain trust and confidence at each level and then move on. Each progressive level of activities brings a new level of satisfaction and self-confidence.

4. **Return Decision-Making Power**

One lady was encouraged to write a list of foods she was not allowed to eat and to keep the card at her bedside to refer to each time a meal was delivered. Consequently, she was more willing to follow dietary restrictions because she felt responsible for correcting the staff on the types of food she should (or should not) be eating.

Other symbols of power include keys, purse, wallet, checkbook with a minimal balance, and pictures of personal possessions. Money can also be used to influence behavior, such as eating healthful foods, exercising, or taking medications. Suggest that it costs much less to stay healthy than it does to seek medical attention. Often, the person makes healthy choices, especially if it saves money.

5. **Provide Positive Reinforcement**

Encourage the person to be proud of accomplishments, even if they has not been done correctly. Treat them in a kind and friendly manner at an appropriate comprehension level. Sometimes a person does

Amira C. Tame, A.C.C.

certain activities because they are comfortable with you, not because they want to do it. If you are good to the person you're caring for, they will pay you back by cooperating, and, eventually enjoying the activity. The difficult step is getting started.

6. **Be Sensitive to Moods and Requests**
   The anxiety and confusion a person with Alzheimer's feels may cause them to pull away from the real world. Consequently, they may regress into depression and cease to communicate or participate in any activity. If you find resistance to all of your attempts to begin productive engagement, you may be able to break the ice with a snack or a cookie.

Remember, for a person with Alzheimer's, activity is anything in which they participate. Eating an apple, a cookie, or a cracker is considered an activity. It does not require physical or mental exercise. Most enjoy ice cream, a special pastry, or chocolate treats. You will likely get a positive response when you get them involved in an activity after just finishing a favorite treat.

Develop Happiness, Enjoyment and Self-Worth

Asking for assistance from a person with Alzheimer's makes them feel important and needed. No one likes to be told what to do or they didn't do something right. In a nonthreatening tone, ask, "Would you like to help cut vegetables? roll pie dough? arrange flowers? decorate a basket? sing a song?" Participation usually increases within a reasonable period of time. As participation in one of these activities becomes routine it becomes easier to increase the level of participation. If you are planning a baking activity and know the person cannot bake, pre-measure the ingredients to eliminate frustration. They can participate in making the baked item and feel a part of its success. It can build self-confidence and be the highlight of the day. This is not simply baking a cake, but participating in a therapeutic activity.

Give the person responsibility to solve or figure something out. Don't always be quick to provide answers for everything. Allow time for independent thoughts. With your encouragement, they can learn to do new things they once thought were impossible. Give them individual tasks to complete. Self-respect is gained by learning to do new things with appropriate activities.

Improve Long and Short-Term Memory

Memory loss is the most obvious effect of Alzheimer's. Although the disease causes progressive deterioration of brain cells, individuals can still utilize available memory capacity and learn new things through specialized activity programs. It is especially rewarding to see persons who were once withdrawn, frightened and lacked enough self-confidence to even speak, finally come "out of their shell" and smile again. Increasing memory base restores self-confidence and self-esteem through selective recall techniques. The Personal Profile Form (see Chapter 3) provides much of this information.

You have probably already discovered most can recall childhood and adolescent periods easier than last week's events. Travel experiences are often remembered in detail. However, instead of asking where they traveled, ask open-ended questions, for example, "Have you ever traveled in the past?" If not, then ask about neighborhood or community events. This may trigger memories of where they traveled, with whom, or other significant events or experiences. They may have worn something special, seen a special show, or eaten exotic foods.

For most of us, food is a resource of many memories associated with cooking, growing, creating food dishes, or eating at special restaurants.

General Techniques

Before meeting with an individual with Alzheimer's, be respectful of their schedule to avoid being viewed as an intruder. With few things in life to enjoy, the last thing you want to do is take any pleasures away. For example, determine when favorite television shows air or what time is best for eating, or what other organized activities are scheduled. The activities will be more successful if they fit within their schedule. When visiting, be sure to respect their home and do not assume they are oblivious of your actions. Do not enter until you have been invited. Always take off your shoes even if you are not asked to. Wait to be invited to sit down, otherwise, you may unknowingly sit in their favorite chair. Smile often and move slowly to prevent triggering anxiety.

A person with Alzheimer's is not always receptive to people entering their room or space. One way to gain entrance is to initially come as a friend of a family member or a companion who is simply stopping by for a visit. This is a nonthreatening approach and usually works. In later stages of the disease, they typically do not want to know you are there for therapeutic purposes. Provide reassurance that you enjoy people and would like to come back as often as possible. Let them know it is no trouble, it is not out of your way at all, and you promise to stop by the next time you are in the area.

It is important for them to express feelings early on. If you ask, "How are you doing?" or "How was your day?," it may cause confusion because it places undue expectations to recall facts or specific events. However, there is no wrong answer for, "How are you feeling today?" Feelings are easier to recall than specific details. Even if the answer is, "I don't know," it is still appropriate. When you ask about feelings, it is heard as a caring question. It provides an opportunity to divulge anything troubling them. If you can understand what is bothering them, you may have the beginning of a successful day. It could be something that has been bothersome for days.

Sharing feelings is the best remedy for healing the wounds of diminished memory function. Keep spirits high by being a good listener and showing you care. Sensing you are listening and paying attention, may help them begin to open up, express thoughts and respond to other stimuli.

It is important for a person in the early stage to understand you can help reduce the negative effects of the disease. By using these therapeutic activities, you can extend or improve their quality of life. Don't wait until the disease affects all areas of one's life. Begin the activities while the greatest benefits can be realized, in the early stage.

Always ask sincere and thoughtful questions. Express interest in feelings instead of facts. Feelings are more personal and promote sharing with someone who cares. Give them an opportunity to express personal sentiments and feelings to you. Show sincerity while listening for responses.

Initially, some feel uncomfortable and do not maintain eye contact while communicating. Ask simple yes or no questions until you reach a subject that shows interest. Build on interest areas to generate more detailed answers and conversation. As you ask progressive-type questions, verbal responses and body language will help you understand his/her comprehension level. Questions that stimulate more detailed answers can be asked once they feel comfortable with you.

Make sure they are not intimidated by your presence. Position yourself at his/her level or slightly lower versus towering over them. Always ask open-ended questions. Always provide and allow for options and choices.

The following sections highlight successful techniques to implement when appropriate:

1. **Curiosity / Interest Arousal**

   One of the main ingredients of successful activities is the ability to arouse curiosity and interest. Information that will help you design activities around past experiences and interests can be found in the **Personal Profile Form** in Chapter 3.

   If you are not getting anywhere as you ask questions, you might say, "Let me tell you a little bit about myself." don't come off as a professional as this may intimidate or frustrate them. Try to be "down to earth" and discuss simple matters. Show an interest in memorable or significant experiences. Physical stimulation will be enhanced if it relates to something significant in the past. For example, a carpenter or contractor may enjoy activities that involve building something simple or measuring a room or fixtures with a tape measure.

   When riding in a car, there are many things you can point out to arouse interest and stimulate conversation. As an example, if you stop at a gas station, ask if they would like to watch you pump gas, wash the windows, or pay the cashier as they wait in the car. Acknowledge attentiveness through eye contact and body language. When you are driving in areas familiar to the person you are caring for, comment on where you are, which direction you are traveling, and your destination.

Try engaging conversation with comments like, "Did you see that crazy driver over there? I hope the police catch him." "Look at that guy over there. Isn't he handsome?" "What a pretty child she is. Do you think she's pretty?" The answer can be a simple yes or no or a more detailed answer. Other questions may include, "Can you see that pretty bird in the tree?" "Do you like that vehicle style? Color?" Though they may not remember anything they've liked, sometimes seeing or trying a once-familiar activity brings back spontaneous memories and sparks a renewed interest in the activity.

2. Motivation Stimulation

Often recall or memory function is not the biggest obstacle to communication. Lack of motivation may be the root problem to overcome. Stimulation to participate in oral or physical activities can be enhanced by suggesting a health-related activity, for example, squeezing a ball for finger/hand exercises.

Asking the person to help you with an activity usually produces an eager response. Persons with Alzheimer's who are parents often helped others in the past and instinctively may agree to help. Once you detect motivation, suggest another activity when they're finished. Emphasize your need to do this activity right away because you are running behind schedule and need help to finish.

Another suggestion is you have tangled yarn or string that you can't untangle on your own.

Placing pictures of favorite foods in the room or placing magazines within sight may encourage eating through subliminal effects.

Never argue or insist with a strong-minded person. Be creative with your approach and make sure you communicate in a positive manner. Be straightforward with your questions and answers. Go with the flow of conversations when necessary to give back some control to the person you're caring for.

Most like to talk about past careers. They feel they were good at what they did and love to share this. Any therapeutic activities even slightly related to a past career are highly recommended because they will typically respond willingly.

Elements for establishing effective communication include:

A. ***Be a good listener***—Good listening skills encourage positive communication and facilitate the opportunity to effectively apply the powerful techniques detailed in this chapter.

Good listening starts with a sincere interest in someone else's feelings and well-being. Be sure to maintain constant eye contact during your conversations. Give assurance that you've heard what is said. Respond with questions or repeat the information. If s/he seems confused, tell them we all feel that way sometimes. Then move on to another subject that you are certain s/he is familiar with or divert attention to a positive and familiar activity.

During conversations, make it clear you not only heard but you understand and can relate. If the person says his/her daughter came to visit, you might say, "That's so nice she came to visit." Ask if it was an enjoyable visit.

B. ***Respond Positively***—Try not to be judgmental of anything they say or do. For example, when responding to word or spelling games, tell them they are a good speller (even if they guessed some wrong answers). When tasks are not performed correctly or things are out of order, always emphasize only the positive outcomes of that activity.

Be as honest as you can without being critical of mistakes or inappropriate actions. Keep a positive response at the tip of your tongue at all times. You may need to use it spontaneously. Always emphasize that they did a good job, no matter how minimal the improvement, if any.

C. ***Reflect compassion and empathy***—If sad feelings are expressed, respond in a manner that shows you understand and have compassion. For example, don't smile or appear amused while listening to a sad event. They are very aware and sensitive to your body language. Allow time to exhaust feelings. Provide empathic responses until it appears appropriate to move to a more positive subject.

If they tell you a story that is supposed to be funny, laugh. Maybe it was the funniest thing you ever heard, and maybe it was not. Be as sincere as possible, but take precautions to preserve the trust that you've developed. Look for positive aspects whenever possible and remind them of the good people they have in their life. Emphasize the positive things they still have to offer.

D. **Show respect**—If a person senses disrespect, they will not likely share anything or want to cooperate. On the other hand, as you continue to show respect, trust will develop. You become a friend, a companion, someone to share things with, to talk to and feel comfortable with.

Remember, some don't realize they have this disease or simply refuse to believe it. Discuss the disease only if it's brought up, or if you are asked to by a primary caregiver.

Always be humble. Never give the appearance of being better, smarter, quicker, or above them in any way. Don't brag about your job. Say as little about your accomplishments as possible in order to stay focused on their issues. The simpler your job description is, the less intimidated and more open they will be to discuss their own life story.

Help out when necessary, and continually show respect. Show respect for the individual's space and feelings, and also his/her body. Some people do not like being touched. Even a gentle or reassuring pat on the hand or arm may be offensive. Be aware of gestures that indicate a preference and respect those wishes.

3. **Attention Diversion**

If the person does not respond or appears uninterested in doing anything, other things may be bothering them. You may be unable to move beyond the negative emotions to determine the problem. Attention diversion is a method to move from this resistive state into a spontaneous and reactive one. A successful diversion is one that prompts attention without encouragement. You can use simple methods like offering a stuffed animal that may have been cuddled at prior sessions. Holding the stuffed animal may stimulate a willingness to participate in other activities.

Spontaneous reading can be prompted by placing favorite magazines or books within eyesight or reach. If they have enjoyed a balloon activity in past sessions, watching you inflate the balloons may stimulate interest in joining you. Look for gestures of anticipation or any reaction indicating a willingness to participate. Body language may tell you when it is time to move on to other activities.

4. **Familiarization by Creative, Repeated Introductions**

Individuals may become comfortable with activities when they can associate them with familiar items. Many games and activities can be created utilizing the familiar items in different activities. They may not even realize why they like particular activities, or may not realize that familiar items are common to favorite games.

Arranging a variety of activities with the same items reduces the number of new tasks or steps to learn, thereby making participation easier. A greater number of activities gives you more useful tools to select from. Plan a variety of activities to monitor progress and select ones you believe will be most beneficial. Don't necessarily select the activity they prefer; instead, encourage new activities first. Try to rotate activities to maintain high interest. There are many ways to use creative repetition to stimulate memories of familiar items. Costume jewelry is fun to use to create a variety of activities. Cover the jewelry items in a bowl of sand to identify. Put the items under coasters and let them guess what is under each coaster. Have them hold the jewelry and tell you whatever thoughts or memories come to mind. They may want to spell the names of the items. If they do well, they can use those names to form sentences.

5. **Increase Enthusiasm Through Positive Encouragement**

This technique encourages individuals with Alzheimer's to try things they thought they could never experience again. Remember, if they even attempt to participate in an activity, it is considered a success. Even showing an effort is an accomplishment and deserves recognition. Some may not openly say it, most are desperate to feel positive and uplifted. Typically, they are aware of diminished abilities and welcome any opportunity to succeed and regain an enthusiasm for life. Often family and/or caregivers are their only hope for feeling good again. Therefore, always try to maintain a positive environment. Make it clear you are a friend who understands and will never give up on helping.

6.   **Communicating at the Appropriate Level**

Studies reflect 93% of communication by individuals with Alzheimer's is nonverbal (body language, eye contact and movements, touching, expressions). This leaves only 7% as spoken communication. Just as any two persons communicating with each other need to speak the same language, so it is with Alzheimer's. The difficulty is determining level of communication that will be effective. With Alzheimer's, you both may speak the same language and still be unable to communicate effectively. Alzheimer sufferers have unique needs, fears, anxieties, and frustrations that affect their ability or willingness to communicate. Combined with the changing levels of memory function and mood swings, communication is a continual challenge. Determining what level of communication works for each person is the first step to communicating at a functional level. Successful communication will enhance the effectiveness of the techniques discussed in this book. Communication with anyone who does not speak at all is possible by effective observation of body language. In fact, many activities don't require oral communication. Often, a smile or gentle gesture indicates what you would like him to do. Listening to soft music will often stimulate gestures that lead to more extensive communication.

7.   **Enticing Them to Participate in Activities**

If they think the activities are in his/her best interest, or will improve their health or memory, they will be more willing to participate. Once convinced of the benefits, doing the activities will provide greater rewards. Observing others in activities and seeing the benefits will encourage the person to participate in activities and for longer periods of time. More importantly, they may be open to try other activities.

Start the activities session slowly. Play favorite music in the background. Start with something relaxing and easy, such as putting beads on a string, peeling potatoes, sorting colored beads. If they are not willing to participate, allow them to watch. Eventually, curiosity will be aroused enough to ask what you are doing. You might say, "I am making a bracelet for my niece's birthday. Would you like to help?" By asking, you are giving them the chance to help you if they want to. Then they can decide whether or not to participate.

The intention is to arouse curiosity about the activity, show it can be done, that it is fun, and encourage participation. Once they decide to do it, be sure not to criticize. Remember to give rewards for participating and always acknowledge an accomplishment, even if it was simply a willingness to attempt to participate.

Treat the individual as an adult at all times. They resent being treated like children.

8. Overcoming Fear of Change

Most typically resist changes for fear of losing what they have. Surroundings have become strange, with a few or no memories of the recent past. There are fewer items in the environment that reflect memories. They try to protect items associated with the memories left. An example is an article of clothing that becomes very important. Possibly it was a gift from a family member, or it has become familiar because it is often worn (a sweater worn each time a chill is in the air). The person may associate this particular sweater with comfort and warmth and does not recall that other sweaters in the closet provide the same warmth. Help them understand that wearing other sweaters is acceptable. Tell them how beautiful the other clothes are. Assure them that the favorite article of clothing will be available to wear on another day. Change is okay!

9. Provide Love, Support, and Friendship

Think of the person you're caring for as a wounded comrade who needs you. Everyone needs love and attention, persons with Alzheimer's are especially desperate for support and friendship. In some ways, they feel guilty for having Alzheimer's and feel undeserving of love and support. Emotionally, they could be starving.

When you realize what this person has lost in life (friends or memories of friends, confidence, familiar skills, the ability to move around independently), you understand how much they need you. Give assurance that you will always be available. Demonstrate your support by always showing respect, and do your best to make them comfortable. Sometimes it is helpful for a family member to remind them about fond memories of events shared together. It is comforting to hear they are remembered for the good things in life. It is helpful to list those events on paper. Sharing the list will validate that you know about their goodness and the success filled life that they enjoyed. Writing a letter detailing how much you care also validates your feelings.

10. Use White Lies as a Diversion Tactic

Though it is not a good idea to tell obvious lies, you should answer questions with positive answers whenever possible. We need to gage behavior and progress considering the effects of Alzheimer's on their mental awareness and stability. Even if the improvement in abilities or behavior is slow, we must continue to encourage them with positive reinforcement.

Always respond with something positive when confronted with a negative situation. If you have negative information you feel you must share, be very sensitive to mood and behavior before deciding the right time, or if it is really in their best interest to have this information. Ask yourself if sharing this information will help avoid hurt feelings by informing them before they find out from someone else, or will knowing only hurt him/her? Sometimes diversions are necessary to avoid confrontational issues or negative feelings.

One client insisted she did not really live in the care facility she was in, but was only visiting and would never want to live in this particular facility. Without disagreeing with her, the caregiver told her she was living there only temporarily and until she felt better, then diverted her attention by asking her to tell her about her home and neighborhood. General questions about what she liked and disliked were also asked. She loved her home and wanted to tell all about it. As a result, she calmed down, relaxed and completely forgot about her original complaint and demand to leave the facility.

11. Be Flexible with Activity Selection

Be aware of responses you receive from your suggestions, and be prepared to hear feedback from the person you're caring for. It is important that before you suggest an activity, you spend some time communicating. Pay close attention to body language and gestures to determine what type of activities may be appropriate. Understanding their mood provides you with an indication of what type of activity will be successful. Don't start right in with an activity without observing receptiveness to the suggestion. Be ready with alternative ideas. If your first attempt fails, be receptive to suggestions about another activity. If what they want to do is acceptable *and* appropriate, it is likely to be more productive. A person with Alzheimer's can be very stubborn when they don't want to do something, so don't look for success at those times. The skill is in finding what they are willing to do and enjoy. While they are doing this activity you can learn more about what they like and dislike. You may find they are not receptive to any mental or organized physical activity, yet would enjoy taking a walk for physical exercise and relaxation. Go with the flow! Don't be confrontational. Accept activities they are willing and able to do today. Tomorrow is a new day and could bring totally different and relatively much better results!

12. Always Give Undivided Attention

Any quality time you spend with your loved one can lead to behavioral improvements. Even on a good day, don't expect every moment to be productive. Expect mood swings to affect the progress of your therapeutic activities. Being aware of these mood swings during a session requires your undivided attention. It may surprise you how aware they are of your attention level. Because attention span is usually short, you must provide the stimulus for continuity during the activities. Persons with Alzheimer's can slip in and out of interest and curiosity in activities easily and frequently.

To maintain interest, try blending one activity into another without a long pause. It may mean you continue to talk or ask questions while you prepare for another activity. Every minute of activity you share can be helpful in some way. Use every available minute of attention, because the next minute may not be meaningful or productive.

13. Encourage Decision-Making Power

Persons with Alzheimer's gradually lose their mental ability to make major decisions. Making decisions is one of the most wonderful characteristics of being a human being and, also, one of the most painful to give up. As the disease progresses, the fear of losing power becomes an obsession. Control of where they live is usually the most difficult to give up. The ability to manage one's home, personal property, and finances are treasured powers, and these losses are very heart-rendering.

Fortunately, we have the ability to restore some of these losses by allowing them to make some of their own day-to-day decisions wherever they can. Giving them choices, when possible, about food, drink, or dress, as well as how to spend time, is an excellent way to revive confidence and self-respect.

They usually will be more cooperative if you ask rather than command. Instead of saying, "It's 2:00 P.M. and time for your lunch. Come and eat," try saying, "I'm feeling somewhat hungry. Would you like to have lunch with me? I enjoy your company." With the second approach, you are inviting rather than bossing, and is more effective.

Keep it simple. Too many choices can be overwhelming. For example, offer two choices of food or drink instead of three. Always present situations or suggestions that allow a yes or no response. For example, "It is a beautiful day. It would be wonderful to breathe some fresh air and enjoy the beautiful garden. Would you like to do that?" Making the decision to go because they may enjoy the beauty of the garden and fresh air, combined with the fact they are making the decision, is much more effective than if you would have said, "Get ready. We are going to take a walk."

Giving people the opportunity to make choices regarding day-to-day activities can be wonderful for reducing mood swings, fear, anxiety and anger.

Not only does the scope of power for persons with Alzheimer's diminish, so does the need for that power. The extent of their need for power becomes limited by the effect of Alzheimer's. Trying to retain power they still have may result in resistant behavior. Maintaining a little power can mean a lot.

New activities are understandably difficult because of fear of failure and lack of confidence in understanding new instructions. It is much easier for a person with Alzheimer's to participate if there is some recollection of the activity. Examples include clipping coupons, tying bows, putting golf balls, playing games, or listening to songs. They may not perform the activity as well as before, but the enjoyment could be even greater today because remembering past experiences is so gratifying. One may recall what a good speller they were when younger, and may believe they still spell as well today. It is important to let them know how good they still are, even when a word is spelled wrong.

Usually they have many positive, rewarding experiences to draw from the past, and it is up to the caregivers to create methods to help draw out as much as possible at each session. With patience

Amira C. Tame, A.C.C.

and perseverance, many useful activities can be enjoyed at any stage of the disease.

14. Introduce New Activities Slowly

The first step in gradual introduction is to talk about an activity and ask questions to obtain an indication of the level of familiarity. During the introduction process, it is important to observe body language and expressions to evaluate his/her willingness to participate. Encourage the person to look at, hold, and talk about what they see and feel when being introduced to new items used in activity.

For example, before you introduce a card game, a person may become familiar with the cards by holding and shuffling the deck, recognizing the numbers, recalling the black and red cards and face cards versus number cards, or that the king is higher than the jack. There are many opportunities with cards to stimulate thinking without playing an actual card game.

Introduce the items in different ways until you find the most effective activity and methodology. When you find an activity the person recalls, don't expect them to recall every detail. A little recognition is usually enough for you to build upon. It may be necessary to begin at the most elementary level and slowly build to more involved participation.

Usually people are more willing to progress to a new level after feeling secure with their current ability. Be sensitive to how well they do with an activity relative to the previous session before increasing the complexity level. Being aware of how much they remember or how quickly they respond provides an indication of when to increase the complexity.

Participation in increasingly more complex activities can elevate satisfaction and confidence level and expand memory base.

As the complexity of the activity increases and the resistance to change is reduced, you are on your way to building positive attitudes and strong relationships. Be willing to change the activity if the person wants to do something else. Before moving on to something new, always let them know how much you enjoyed the current activity.

15. Begin with Simple Responses

Reflex responses, the most basic type of physical activity, are defined as spontaneous gestures or actions that appear to be involuntary and unplanned. It is beneficial to understand some of the reflex techniques you can use to encourage participation in an activity. Reflex responses effectively provide transition from a passive activity (listening or watching) to active participation.

Reflex reactions can be stimulated by natural survival or neurological stimuli. A balloon gently "bumped" in the air will usually result in a response to "bump" it back to you or catch it as it comes toward him/her. Try to make him/her comfortable with the object before eliciting these types of responses. Another activity is rolling a foam ball.

After touching the ball, feeling how soft it is, and determining it will not hurt, s/he will very likely kick it back. If the ball is not returned, ask them to help you retrieve it. A soft ball held in the palm may generate a squeezing activity which could be considered a conditioned response with a relaxing effect. Music or singing can result in spontaneous foot or hand tapping, humming, dancing or other body movements. If they are physically unable to dance, memories of the times when they could dance may result in an upbeat attitude and stimulate conversation.

16. Select Activities that can be Modified as Skills Improve

Activities that are modified to their level will help maintain interest and are useful in building self-confidence and continuity between skill levels. It is useful for them to learn a new activity on the same level of ability. When they are comfortable with the activities, a higher level can be tried. As their ability changes, progress can be measured by adjusting skill level for the same activity. Improved memory function can be observed after repeated exposure to familiar activities. Introducing creative skill progression can provide the variety necessary to maintain interest.

Dominos is an example of a game that can be customized for progressive skill levels as follows:

- holding or stacking the pieces
- turning the pieces to see the dots
- counting the dots on each piece
- matching the number of dots with other pieces
- recognizing the number and spelling it
- turning a piece face down and recalling the number of dots
- playing a complete game of dominos

Most familiar games or activities can be adjusted to various achievement levels. Don't be discouraged if they can't play cards as before. Break the game down into its basic parts. It may have to begin by recognizing the game, pieces, or numbers. Asking them to help you with the game sometimes reduces fear.

Each of the activities described in this book can be broken down into varying levels of participation. For each activity, determine at which skill level the person's abilities fit, and then design activities so s/he can progress to a higher skill level. Your goal is to involve them as much as possible. Let them enjoy the activity, and whenever appropriate, promote advancement to a higher level of activity and self-confidence.

17. Reward Achievements

Emotional rewards usually are very helpful in gaining acceptance and respect. Recognition for accomplishments provides motivation to improve during the next session or activity. Remember, as the disease progresses, feelings of accomplishment and self-worth diminish. A reward provides an incentive to participate in an activity. As a result, self-confidence and trust in you will grow stronger. Rewards also provide a sense of accomplishment for the caregiver when you can offer recognition for noticeable improvement.

Give praise for accomplishments and let family members know what those accomplishments are so they can help continue the progress. Explain the significance of each improvement. It's not what you say, but what s/he believes. Even if the improvement was slight, it merits recognition from everyone. Knowing there is some measure of improvement can be the motivation necessary to sustain positive relationships with loved ones.

18. Humor Therapy

"Laughter is the closest distance between two people." (Victor Borge)

Sometimes the only way to deal with stress is to find humor in one's situation. When it comes to dealing with Alzheimer's disease, a smile often works better than words. Humor and light-heartedness are often the best medicine for the stress the disease brings to you and the person you're caring for.

With Alzheimer's disease, it's not easy to find something to laugh about in an environment surrounded by clouded memories and diminishing physical abilities. Humor can be most effective if it is injected into an activity session without them being aware of your intent. You cannot hold tension and laugh at the same time.

For my friend with Alzheimer's, laughing didn't take away his condition, but you are able to laugh . . . when he could turn to me and laugh about his situation, it was relief for both of us.

By opening up and giving permission to play and enjoy your loved one, both of you can find plenty of laughter as you indulge in the lighter side of what can be a difficult burden.

Often, persons with Alzheimer's can recall their early childhood more clearly than they can more recent events. If you share some of your humorous childhood memories, they may laugh with you, and more importantly it may trigger their own funny experiences they are willing to share with you. They usually know they have difficulty remembering things, so recalling anything from their past is reassuring and encourages participation in other activities.

"There ain't much fun in medicine, but there is a lot of medicine in fun." *Josh Billings)*

"Humor is the instinct for taking pain playfully." *(Mark Eastman)*

"I would never have made it if I could not have laughed. Laughing lifted me momentarily . . . out of this horrible situation, just enough to make it livable . . . survivable." (Victor Frankl)

"This I believe to be the chemical function of humor: to change the character of our thought." (Lin Yutang)

"The chemicals that are running our body and our brain are the same chemicals that are involved in emotion. And that says to me that . . . we'd better pay more attention to emotions with respect to health." *(Candace Pert)*

"A clown is like an aspirin, only he works twice as fast."

Minimizing Resistant Behavior

Resistant behavior often results in resistant conversation. Without verbal communication, it is difficult to understand what is troubling the person you're caring for. They have mood swings just like anyone else, and hardly says a word, and make it very difficult to move forward. Often the real issues at hand can be determined by using information shared and interacting with family members.

Once the individual opens up, listen carefully and go with the flow. Use this opportunity to assess any needs or wants. Respond immediately, if possible, to any request that you can help with. Show you are not only listening but you also care. The reward is that they feel better and appreciate the fact that you understood his/her needs and were able and happy to fulfill them. It reduces any feeling of guilt when you know you've done what you can to please someone who really needs your help.

Techniques to Minimize Resistant Behavior Include:

- Encourage participation at his/her level of competence and capability.
- Use passive activities to stimulate a response.
- Ask for assistance with things you know they enjoy.
- Allow them to watch you do an activity without asking them to participate.
- Avoid discussing difficult or sensitive issues (finances, property, politics, religion, or disliked friends/family).
- Some may or may not want to talk about Alzheimer's disease, so be sensitive to their wishes.
- If finances are brought up, discuss them in a manner so they feel secure and not confronted or threatened.

Additional Hints for Minimizing Resistant Behavior Include:

- Wearing brightly colored clothes often lifts spirits and mood. According to the American Institute for Biosocial Research, "colors are electromagnetic wave bands of energy." Stimulated by colors, glandular activities can alter moods, speed up heart rates, and increase brain activity. Most seem to enjoy brightly-colored pictures. Men seem to prefer blue, and women like orange, pink, and red. Both sexes like pictures of animals and flowers, especially yellow or blue flowers and green plants. Pictures of flower gardens often spark comments about how they used to plant or gather such flowers. Happiness reflects in their faces, eyes light up, and smiles break out.
- As a caregiver, you might be the only "bright spot" in the person's life, and whether you portray positiveness or negativeness, it will likely be reflected in their attitude.
- Attractively styled hair and makeup tastefully applied shows that you respect yourself and the person you're caring for. We show respect to others when our appearance is at its best. They deserve and crave as much respect as you can give them because theirs has been eroded by this disease.
- The caregiver has to consider the Alzheimer's disease challenge as being twofold—the individual and the disease. Sometimes the caregiver is frustrated and angry with the individual. It is difficult to remember that this problem was not caused by the

person suffering from Alzheimer's. What you are remembering is a different person—loving, caring, helpful, active, and having a good memory. If you want to truly help now, you must help fight the disease, not the person. Look at the individual as your team member, sharing your goals and activities. Treat him/her the way you would like to be treated if you needed the same help.

- Share your other daily experiences in simple (not childish) terms. Share what is going on in your life, where you've been today, what your plans are for the rest of the day, or whom you have seen. They love to hear these stories and share your experiences with you on an adult basis, like a friend.
- The focus of these initial low-level activities is to stimulate conversation channels and show genuine interest in their likes and dislikes. This must be done in a nonthreatening and simple fashion and be based on opinions and feelings and not facts. Ask questions for which there can be no wrong answers, no matter what the response. Questions that can be answered by a simple yes or no are ideal.

Summary

Any activity can be helpful by the way you present it. Helping you do something that they would not do for themselves (coloring Easter eggs for church, club, or grandchildren) will give them a feeling of giving back. All of these activities enhance the mental goals of this book. One of the most important goals is to improve overall mental and physical capabilities. It is up to the caregiver to decide which methodologies will work best.

Preparing for Activities

1. Make sure that the activity you choose considers all of the guidelines and information in the Personal Profile Form (Chapter 3).

Rescue Activities

The following are rescue activities you can resort to when the person you're caring for does not feel like participating in any activities, or is not in a good mood:

- Eating ice cream, cookies, cakes, or favorite fruits or drinks
- Walking in a garden, on the sidewalk, in the mall, or a favorite place
- Going shopping
- Watching favorite TV shows/programs, movies
- Watching a favorite game, sport or exercise show can involve them in an activity without participating
- Visiting with live or stuffed animals can provide companionship (watching or feeding birds can be relaxing)

General Guidelines

In choosing an activity, the main goal is for it to be successful—nothing else matters. Therefore, choose activities based on the person's abilities to participate and handle. For example, a person with later stage Alzheimer's can participate in a card game by just watching other people playing, or can sort the cards by colors or numbers, etc. Eventually they may be able to participate in more complicated activities, including playing simple card-matching games, such as Old Maid, Fish, War, etc.

Food Area—adjust the food related activities to their ability to participate. In later stages, just eating their favorite meal at home, or watching a TV show on food, snack or dessert preparation may be the level of activity that is appropriate. In earlier stages, involving them in preparing and cooking the food (sorting, washing, cutting) may be appropriate.

Writing the recipe in large letters and in simple steps will make it easier to read and understand and will reduce the chance of embarrassment or humiliation. If possible, use familiar recipes. This helps them complete the steps with confidence.

Caution: be careful not to let them use tools, such as a sharp knife, they might hurt themselves with.

- Introduce activities slowly and in a non-threatening manner. Involve them in deciding what activity they will be participating in.
- Present activities in a goal-oriented and helpful manner. Example: "My cousin's birthday is tomorrow and I have to bake her a cake

Amira C. Tame, A.C.C.

and I am short on time. Would you help me so I can finish it? It will mean a lot to her". Agreeing to help does not make them responsible for finishing and completing the mission by themselves and possibly failing to do it right. Don't insist that they help, but if they do choose to help it can be a very beneficial activity. They often enjoy helping you do something needed (sorting cards to put them away, sorting sewing to make it neat so you can easily find what you are looking for).

- Allowing them to do one step at a time will result in a successful activity. Any steps they help you with will be considered successful.
- Many times successful activities can be built around their experiences, including work, hobbies, and vacations, etc. A professional painter would most likely still enjoy painting or using painting tools in their activities. Give them the opportunity to paint small items, for example, a wood model home, model car, mailbox, bird house, dog house, etc. Protect the area for a painting activity with plastic covers on the floor and table; use washable paint; and provide a large shirt or smock to wear over regular clothes.
- Ask someone with a familiar background to visit with the person you're caring for. They might enjoy this new visitor who has a background that they can identify with, and it may stimulate memories of their working relationship. Many people are happy to volunteer time to visit and help out. Family members, friends, neighbors, or local churches are helpful resources for finding an appropriate visitor. This information is included in their Personal Profile Form (Chapter 3).

Chapter 5

Resolving Physical and Functional Issues

Now that you . . .

. . . understand the effects of Alzheimer's disease (Chap. 1)

. . . have learned how caregivers can reduce feelings of anger, frustration, and helplessness (Chap. 2)

. . . have learned as much as you can about the person with Alzheimer's, including historical and current data (Chap. 3)

. . . are familiar with the effective methods and techniques to treat the symptoms of Alzheimer's disease (Chap. 4)

You are ready to . . .

. . . begin the healing process!

Amira C. Tame, A.C.C.

Understanding the Healing Process

The healing process must begin by removing communication obstacles. Only when there is effective communication can progress be made in other areas.

Obstacles to communication may be caused by preexisting physical conditions. Some of these conditions can be resolved by providing necessary implements or aids. It is also important, however, to understand some impairments are permanent. These may be either physical or mental impairments that are not expected to improve.

This chapter is dedicated to removing the obstacles you can do something about improving your relationship with the person you are caring for. Many of the issues addressed in this chapter can be resolved by discovering and eliminating the underlying root causes using resourceful intervention techniques. Other issues can be resolved through the use of customized activities described in Chapter 6.

The goal is to see them do more and you do less. This removes some of the burden for you to do everything and is considered a win-win situation because it enhances the quality of life for both of you. Hopefully, there will be less frustration and decreased stress levels.

Understanding the effects of Alzheimer's makes it easier to identify the behavioral and other difficulties you are faced with daily as you care for a person suffering with this disease. Similar to other challenges, you must define the specific issues, decide which ones you would like to improve, determine root causes, and finally, design a therapeutic activity program to achieve the desired results.

During the survey process, you gathered important information to identify and establish the scope of the issues (what are the issues, the severity, and who is affected). The next step is to determine which issues are physical difficulties that can be resolved by physical means. You must be aware of any physical impairments when designing activities.

Any physical aids or devices normally used must always be available to decrease discomfort. Often, they are unable to express the source of discomfort (e.g., pain, nausea or constipation). Thus it is important to determine whether the problem is caused by a sensory impairment (sight, hearing, taste or touch) or a physical impairment (paralysis, arthritis, etc.). Look for body language that indicates problems not clearly obvious.

The first phase of healing is designed to reduce physical and functional issues that hinder communication and cause negative feelings and alienation. Successfully implemented, this phase significantly enhances the mental and physical well-being and prepares him/her for the second phase, detailed in Chapter 6. This phase details customized activities designed to continually improve memory function, physical ability, and overall emotional well-being.

The purpose of discussing how to resolve physical and functional issues before engaging in activity therapy is twofold. First, it is important to emphasize the removal of as many distractions and obstacles as possible. Attention span and motivation are generally diminished to the extent that any obstacle will hinder participation in an activity. The second reason is to ensure your expectations are realistic and will lead to an improved quality of life for both you. Leave open the possibility that any issue may have a cause secondary to Alzheimer's disease. Always keep an open mind as you proceed through the remaining chapters.

Getting Started

Understanding the effects of Alzheimer's disease makes it easier to identify the behavioral and other difficulties you are faced with daily. The first important step is to define the specific issues.

Issues that affect the quality of life for all persons affected by this disease typically fall into one or more of the following categories:

Physical/Functional

Hearing
Sight
Eating
Mobility
Personal Appearance/Hygiene

Cognitive

Daily Tasks and Routines

Behavioral/Emotional

Attention
Anger
Isolation
Resistance and Attachment
Personal Possessions/Trust

Environmental

Wandering
Adapting to Facility or Home
Being Disruptive

Prioritize Goals

Decide which issues, if resolved, would provide the greatest benefits for everyone. Although you may want to target everything, select one or two so it is easier to focus on improvements. Most likely whenever you are making progress on some issues, your activities are having a positive effect on others. It is important to continually review the Client Intake Goals / Assessment Report and Activities Progress Report in Chapter 3.

How to Identify Root Causes

The first step in identifying the root cause of a problem is to eliminate the possibility that it is a pre-existing condition not likely to change, as identified in the Personal Profile Form (completed in Chapter 3). Next, narrow down the possibilities by answering the following questions:

- Where does the problem occur? Are they having difficulty while in the dining room, lounge, bed, alone or in the presence of someone?
- When does the problem occur? Morning, afternoon, evening, before meals, after meals?

- What are they doing when the problem occurs? Dressing, watching television, eating, walking, participating in an activity?

If it is during an activity, possibly the activity level is too stressful for their ability.

- Who is near or interacting when the problem occurs? The same person, a group, a certain visitor, caregiver, aide, nurse, or the activity therapist?
- Is the physical problem actually a physical issue?
- Do others in the facility or home express a similar problem?
- Was the problem evident prior to Alzheimer's?
- What changes may have intensified the problem?

Resolving Physical and Functional Issues

Physical and functional issues can be the root cause of apparent behavioral problems, although the individual may not be aware of the sources of his/her irritation or discomfort. Helping remove these obstacles will pave the way for you to address the issues caused by Alzheimer's disease.

Hearing

Reduced hearing capabilities cause an inability to hear instructions which, in turn, is often interpreted as resistant behavior. Inability to hear the television or radio, unless the volume is turned so high that others are disturbed, often creates animosity with others who dislike loud noise. The problem can usually be easily overcome with the use of a hearing aid (or turning up the one s/he has and/or checking the battery), ear phones, or head phones to listen to favorite programs. This helps to reduce anxiety, overcome communication obstacles, and restore enjoyment of favorite pastimes.

Being able to hear what is said is the other half of communication. As difficult as it is to cope with the challenges and realities of Alzheimer's disease, do not forget the many other effects of aging that something *can* be done about. If there is still difficulty hearing, speak loudly, slowly, and directly so s/he can see your lips move. Offer written instructions if they can read.

Seeing

Difficulty in seeing might be resolved by simply getting new glasses or asking them to wear the pair s/he already has. Communication by sight is often hampered by age-related disorders that can be overcome by providing large print books, audio books, large screen television (closed-caption if hearing impaired), oversized telephone numbers (one-touch dialing if unable to comprehend numbers), or large numbered clocks. The feeling of being able to see and hear better as a result of your assistance encourages cooperation and trust when you introduce therapeutic activities.

Eating

Eating difficulties may be a result of improper fitting or missing dentures, sore and painful gums, periodontal diseases, or abscessed teeth. Sometimes an eating difficulty is misinterpreted as resistant behavior when in reality it is an acquired dislike for certain foods or a result of reduced sensory response to particular flavors. Try enhancing the taste by adding salt, salt substitutes or a spice appropriate for that particular dish. With sweetened foods, try sugar, sugar substitutes, honey, or sugar-free sweeteners.

If enhancing the flavors does not work, it may be necessary to change the diet slightly or completely. Also check the side effects of prescribed medications to determine if appetite or food taste can be affected. If so, ask the medical doctor to consider another medication. Hopefully, your persistence will result in better eating habits. You could also try customizing reading activities to include pictures and articles about foods. Looking at pictures of prepared food may stimulate interest in a new dish or rekindle a memory of a favorite dish from the past.

Leave behind food magazines and pictures so s/he can read or browse at any time. Pictures of fruit baskets or cut fruits can be stimulating and encourage eating. Remind them about the benefits of eating well. One effective motivator to staying healthy is the fact it costs less to be healthy than to be sick. A simple reminder that his/her money will be spent on doctors and health care if s/he gets sick may promote better eating habits and increased exercise to stay healthy and save money.

Mobility

Test physical impairments to determine whether they are truly physical or possibly psychological in nature, and also to determine the root cause of the issue. Some impairments caused by lack of physical stimulus can be identified through exercise activities that target the impairments. The root cause of apparent physical challenges are sometimes mentally induced.

Case Study:

> *An example of a mentally-induced physical problem is illustrated by a 79-year-old client of mine who never used her left arm. When I asked family and staff members, I was told she lost the use of her left arm some time ago. It could not be established that this condition was caused by any traumatic injury or stroke, etc. It was important for me to know if there was any hope for her ever being able to use her left arm so I could design my activities accordingly. I decided to try a balloon toss activity that hopefully would stimulate a spontaneous reactive response. The object of the activity was to bump the balloon back to me each time I tossed it toward her. After repeatedly tossing the balloon to her right side until her response became automatic, I quickly switched to her left side, and to my amazement, she spontaneously used her left hand to bump it back. I continued to switch back and forth and she continued to use both arms. After the activity ended, I calmly asked if her left arm felt better, and she said yes. I was so thrilled I could hardly wait to tell her family. After that, she stopped tucking her left arm tightly to her side as though it were immobile. She simply forgot that it didn't work.*

A person who sits in one chair all day or in bed most of the time may not feel confident or capable of moving around. Maybe a new walker or wheelchair is needed to regain mobility, but s/he is unable to express this. You may need to walk alongside to provide a feeling of security and self-confidence. It is possible their shoes do not fit anymore or are worn to one side, causing pain or unstable walking. They may not be unable to say what hurts or doesn't work, so it is up to you to be aware of actions and body language when they respond to your requests. Look for a grimace or other physically spontaneous reactions that could indicate a physical rather than an emotional cause.

In many instances, as a caregiver you are an extension of their sensory perceptions, his/her mouthpiece to express feelings, and his/her lifeline to obtaining assistance. Finding help for any of the physical difficulties will begin building the relationship between you and the individual you're caring for. S/he will soon discover you care enough to help.

Personal Appearance / Hygiene

Resistance to changing clothes is a common problem among persons with Alzheimer's. Many forget there are other clothes to wear. It is possible s/he has narrowed his/her taste in clothes to one item. After all, it is one less decision that needs to be made each day, and with a diminishing memory capacity, this could be a mental coping method to conserve available memory. Unfortunately, if they are looking for an easy way out, it is easy to get in a rut. His/her mind won't be challenged to increase memory capacity.

Encourage Variety in Dress

There are things you can do to encourage variety dressing. Once you have observed a particular outfit in the closet, compliment them about how nice s/he looked wearing this outfit in the past. Look in the closet and praise his/her good taste in clothes. If you know who purchased the clothes, comment how nice it was of that person to do so. Noting a special occasion when an outfit was worn might inspire them to try it on again. Convince him/her the clothes being worn now need to be laundered to look cleaner and last longer.

As a last resort, if they repeatedly ask for a particular article of clothing, state that a spot didn't come out, the article needed to be replaced because it was too old, or it is at the dry cleaner and will be a little while longer before it is cleaned. If there is nothing else in the closet they like, offer to take them on a shopping trip to select a new outfit. Hopefully this will be viewed as a fun and positive experience.

Help them Choose

Make sure the colors and materials are his/her favorites. Don't ask them to wear a wool sweater that might feel irritating. Also, be certain the temperature in the home is considered when selecting an outfit. If they continue to resist changing clothes regularly, it could be the dressing methods are confusing and s/he is wearing the clothes easiest to put on. Suggest shopping for new clothes that are easy to dress with, e.g., wraparounds, snaps or zippers (buttons are usually harder). Most importantly, be consistent in order to minimize confusion. Observe them dressing and determine if it is difficult to decide what to wear or to dress once the article is chosen. If they are still having a hard time dressing, help him/her dress or ask someone else to help.

Standing in front of the closet with 25+ outfits and expecting them to choose is simply too overwhelming. If selection is the issue and s/he seems willing to choose something else, but can't decide easily, try minimizing the choices by telling what your favorite two are, or ask if you could help by putting tags on each hanger to indicate when a particular outfit is to be worn. This still gives them a choice without having to be frustrated with a daily decision of what to wear.

Resolving Cognitive Issues

Now that you have identified and resolved physical and functional issues, you have instilled a sense of confidence that will continue to improve their quality of life.

They are probably already feeling better knowing you are their advocate and someone who cares about their well-being. It will thus be much easier to move on to activities that address cognitive and behavioral issues.

Orientation and Familiarization

We want them to be as independent and self-reliant as possible. Remember, our goal is to increase their level of independence. You must develop methods to ease the difficulty so they can do as many personal tasks as possible.

Amira C. Tame, A.C.C.

Helping to organize daily routines to make it easier to find bedrooms, lunchrooms, or bathrooms with signs or colored tape reduces stress and allows them to manage necessary daily functions. A flip-type daily calendar showing only one date at a time may be effective in reducing confusion.

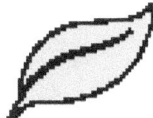 *Cognitive issues can be minimized by recognizing the affected functions and adjusting the environment to accommodate the difficulties encountered.*

Cognitive issues can be minimized by recognizing the affected functions and adjusting the environment to accommodate the difficulties encountered. Loss of memory function can be frustrating when it affects basic necessities such as moving around the house, finding the bathroom, using the telephone, remembering telephone numbers, going to the kitchen, finding the bedroom, getting dressed, bathing. When these difficulties pile up, frustration can turn into depression, anger, or violence.

They may be too vain to admit forgetting where to go. Help to eliminate this problem by putting signs and arrows on doors and walls showing how to get around the house. Signs leading to his/her bedroom will help provide direction as s/he comes and goes within the home. Put colored arrows along the bottom of the wall or on the floor that lead to the areas s/he can't get to independently. Provide notes indicating what color to follow to get to certain rooms. This technique reduces frustration and provides a sense of independence.

Some refuse to bathe, shower, comb hair, or brush teeth. Loss of memory function may have affected the ability to even recognize what a toothbrush is used for.

Some have been observed trying to shave with a toothbrush. Some look in the mirror and think it is someone else. Try putting a note on the mirror that says: "Mom, this is you in the mirror." This simple note may help to explain why the person in the mirror didn't answer when spoken to.

Often they don't recognize themselves. If they are afraid of getting into the bathtub, there could be a fear of slipping and falling. A rubberized mat or a stool to sit on will help reduce this fear. Fear of a shower could stem from early childhood experiences when only a bathtub was available. Infrequent showering could also be a result of a family environment in that it was not possible to bathe each day. A hand-held shower adapter with an on/off switch may help by providing more control and reduce their fear.

Wandering

In the early stage of Alzheimer's some feel they don't belong in a facility or think they can still drive a car well. In fact, those who have retained communication skills appear unaffected by the disease. Until you are with them long enough to observe the symptoms first hand, you too might also question why they are there. Some want to leave so strongly that, when left unattended, they walk away from the home or facility.

Remind them that there is a contract agreement to remain at the care facility for a period of time and it would be a waste of money to leave before the contract is up. They promised to honor this agreement and not fight the decision to stay. Most do not want to look bad and will try to be responsible and stand behind the agreement. Remind them that staying is in their best interest. The caregiver and the rest of the family have many other obligations (children, careers and homes), and if they remain willingly at the center, it is easier for everyone.

Be careful not to hurt their feelings. Continually remind them of your care and concern and that they are missed while away. Share how you feel with staff members who work at the facility so they can continually reinforce your commitment to them in case the desire to leave is mentioned.

Limit walks alone to an enclosed area or within sight of a caregiver. Longer walks must be supervised at all times.

In later stages of the disease, individuals can easily get lost while going for a walk. Sometimes, as soon as they leave their environment. Knowing that they have agreed to a contract to stay at the facility and how much you care about them will provide the motivation to stay.

Behavioral / Emotional

The source of problems or issues is not always obvious. Often, behavioral issues are caused by something not connected with the issue at all. As you try to comfort a person who is anxious or disruptive, observe body language that may indicate what is causing the unacceptable behavior. Resolving some of the physical, functional and cognitive issues has probably resulted in behavioral improvement. Removing the obstacles to performing daily functions independently has probably reduced stress and anxiety levels and enhanced the likelihood of a successful activities program. Similar to physical and functional issues, you can often discover root causes for many behavioral issues. Try to determine if the behavioral issues have roots other than emotional ones.

Anger

Anger that has escalated to violent behavior is the most difficult barrier to overcome. While you are seeking root causes for behavioral issues, you still need to cope with the symptoms and reduce the intensity as much as possible to establish communication. Effective communication is virtually impossible at a high level of anger.

Ron, most of the time, has good behavior. On one occasion, he suddenly grabbed me by my arm. He was a very large man and very strong. I was scared. He told me to come with him as he tightened his grip on my arm, and led me down the hallway leading to the residents' rooms. I said, "Ron, I'm happy to come with you." I knew that if I resisted, his violence would escalate, and he might hurt me. He led me from one resident's room to another, insisting that I open each door. I gladly obliged. My cool response to this potentially dangerous situation provided the staff time to recognize the situation and call for help. Help did arrive to diffuse the situation and provide Ron with the assistance he needed.

It is very difficult for a person to become interested in or even think about an activity if the overriding emotion is anger. When the anger has no outlet, it can become a violent outburst resulting in hitting and yelling. As a caregiver, it is imperative to maintain a cool composure and not let the angry feelings transfer to you. You can't fight fire with fire. If they strike out, don't take it personally. At that moment, s/he may not even know who you are or what is being said. Tell them that it hurts when s/he strikes out and ask them to not do it again. Say it is okay to feel angry and you would like to help them feel better. Emphasize the time you spend together is special and you enjoy taking time to visit. Try to divert attention from whatever is causing the negative behavior.

Almost all individuals enjoy ice cream or cookies and will respond positively if you politely ask if s/he would like to join you. Sugar free and low-fat options are available at most ice cream shops. Yogurt ice cream is also a good choice for some. At some stage, eating out of a cup may be easier to manage. When they see you eating or enjoying something you are doing, s/he may want to share that enjoyment with you. Keep a positive attitude and, whenever possible, encourage him/her to do something enjoyable. This may help to reduce frustration and anxiety.

If the aggressiveness remains at a high level and there is still a significant amount of resistance, curtail your attempts and observe his/her behavior from a distance to give time to respond or calm down quietly.

Anger with parents could be a way to externalize the fact s/he has the disease, i.e., "It's not my fault I have this problem—it must have been passed on by my mother or father," or from a distant relative who had the same symptoms.

Isolation

Another symptom of anger can manifest itself in antisocial behavior or isolation, and if not resolved, can lead to complete withdrawal. This is an emotional issue that is much easier to resolve than anger and violence.

Withdrawal is not always caused by anger. A combination of emotional changes that occur with Alzheimer's disease may be causing the withdrawal. Or it could be a feeling of not belonging and not fitting in. Fear of being unable to find the right words when speaking causes them to withdraw into a shell with no hope of coming out. Without your help, they may feel more and more alienated from friends and family and these negative feelings will become an obstacle to productive engagement. Make them feel increasingly more useful.

It is likely that a person who was easily angered before having Alzheimer's can still be easily angered and hostile. The same applies to a previously introverted person who pulls into a shell more easily and prefers passive activities. It is important to understand what type of personality the person had before the disease in order to determine his/her potential for improvement. The Personal Profile Form Form (Chapter 3) provides an idea of the extent the disease has affected his/her behavior. Pain and depression can also cause isolation and hostile behavior.

It is easy to see why completing the root cause analysis is necessary to uncover the real cause of the outwardly expressed behavioral symptoms.

Isolation can be so severe that they won't even leave a chair or couch without resistant or disruptive behavior. Try to establish a relationship without requiring them to move. Engage in constructive conversation where they are. A pleasant atmosphere can have a calming effect on a distressed person. While they are relaxing may be a good time to share personal information if you are a family member. They may enjoy hearing things forgotten or something they've not heard before. It might encourage them to share things with you.

Attachment

When you are finally able to coax a withdrawn person out of their room and they begin to enjoy being out, you may encounter resistance when it is time to return to the room. Going back to the room could be a signal you will be leaving soon and they may want to prolong your stay. Allow time for more activities after you return to their room to reduce the possibility of separation anxiety. Reassure them you will be back soon. If you have a specific visitation day, mark it on a calendar for him/her to see. This will serve as a reminder of your next meeting and also lends credibility to what you've promised. It is easier to believe you will return if they see it written down.

Resistance to Taking Medication

Try to find out the root cause of resistance to taking medication. Maybe the medication tastes bad and needs to be mixed with food or liquid. It is possible they don't trust the person providing the medication or is afraid the prescription may be wrong. If possible, show the order from the doctor or their name on the bottle.

Another possible cause is an adverse reaction or side effects that they are unable to understand or express. Make sure you understand which side effects to look for as a possible cause for rejection. If you notice any, inform the staff or the family doctor. It may be possible to prescribe an alternative medicine without side effects. If the root cause is mistrust of the person providing the medication, find someone else to provide the medication. If they mistrust everyone, it may be necessary to put medications in food or drinks.

Mistrust and Misunderstanding

Mistrust of the person caring for their personal belongings can be especially frustrating and unsettling. Material possessions may be the only security they have to hold on to. With their memory becoming progressively less reliable, even these possessions are now at risk of being lost. Not knowing the whereabouts or destiny of possessions can result in mistrust of those people who are helping care for them.

Relocation

As the disease progresses, it may be necessary to seek closer supervision and may require relocation to a care facility. Understandably, this could be very disconcerting. Usually one's home is a revered possession with a strong connection to ownership. It is usually the most costly possession in a person's life. No one looks forward to being incapable of maintaining a home or making decisions about personal destiny.

Reassure them the decision to move is a good one. Money received from the sale of the home will pay for the special care s/he deserves. Assure them you will be much more comfortable knowing they are always around others in case of an emergency.

Assure them your visits will be more enjoyable if you don't have to waste time talking about how much you worry about them, and you'll have much more time to share.

If they are no longer able to drive, indicate you are available for errands. Say, "I'll take you wherever you need to go. I worry when you drive and I'm afraid you might hurt someone else, too. I'll take you anywhere, anytime, and it will be an opportunity for us to spend time together. If you'd like, I can drive your car when we go. It's better for a car to be driven instead of sitting in one place. Maybe you'd like to sell it to 'a family member'

Amira C. Tame, A.C.C.

to keep it in the family. If you would rather keep it, we can park it in the garage until you are able to use it."

Money Issues

Knowing their money or financial holdings are safe gives them a sense of security. Confirm that all bank accounts are secure. Show bank statements, if possible, to confirm the status of the accounts. Money provides a sense of power. Without the assurance that their money is safe, they may feel trapped and out of control. Always make sure they have money to give them a feeling of security in case something needs to be purchased. Even if there is no way to spend money, provide a few dollars just for the feeling of security. If you are concerned they might lose or misplace the money, it's a small price to pay for the security and sense of power it provides. If the money is lost, don't make an issue of it. Simply replace it and try to find a secure place to keep it. If you are the primary caregiver and you are going away for an extended period of time, provide reassurance you've left money in the staff office or with a trusted relative. When possible, take them with you to the bank to see their money is safe. Let them ask the teller questions if they wish.

Environment

Try to create the most stable and safe environment possible, given the circumstances. This period in their life is filled with uncertainty. Moving personal belongings in the room can be very distressing to someone suffering from memory loss. Moving even one item can possibly cause confusion and create suspicion that something is missing, or they are in the wrong room.

If possible, try to furnish the room with familiar fixtures and furniture. If they live at home, refrain from rearranging or replacing furniture. If it is necessary to move to a care facility, take personal furniture there to help them be more comfortable. It takes a long time for someone suffering from Alzheimer's disease to adjust to a new environment, and they most certainly will be confused if there continues to be too many changes. Individuals with Alzheimer's grasp for any stability they can find. New and unfamiliar items cause confusion and frustration.

Personal Property

Memory loss also affects the perception of what belongs to them and what doesn't. Sometimes this results in property belonging to one person being taken by another, creating a difficult and embarrassing situation for you as a caregiver and a potentially upsetting outcome.

Don't overreact when this happens. Once you have determined the property is in the wrong hands, simply try to return it to the rightful owner without fanfare. Treat them with respect because more than likely it was an unintentional act without malice or conscious intent. Don't grab the item. Ask if s/he minds if you return the item to the original owner because that person probably needs and misses it. If you encounter resistance, try to ignore the situation for a short time. Move on to something else and pay close attention to where the person keeps or hides it. When you have an opportunity, take the property back and try not to expose the item to them again, if possible.

Monitor the Progress

Use the Personal Profile Form, Client Intake Goals—Assessment Report, and Activities Progress Report (Chapter 3) as tools to track your progress. Often it is easy to recognize if your approach is working by observing immediate responses, but some improvements take longer and are not as pronounced as others. Perform a self-assessment after two months of working toward your goals to determine if negative-type incidents have been reduced, or if memory appears to have been improved. Continue measuring progress, whether positive or negative, throughout your activity program.

Sundowners Syndrome

Sundowning, or "sundowners syndrome" is a condition that occurs later in the day. It is a symptom and not a condition itself, nor a separate disease.

Many symptoms of Alzheimer's disease are more apparent in the late afternoon and evening hours. Evening is the most challenging time of the day for caregivers.

- Fear
- Depression
- Confusion
- Agitation
- Uncooperative behavior
- Nonparticipation in activities
- Anger
- Hallucination
- Restlessness
- Sleeplessness

What causes Sundowners Syndrome?

There are many physical reasons, e.g. reaction to medication, pain, hunger, need to urinate, fatigue, uncomfortable clothes etc. that cause a person to have Sundowner symptoms. It is not clear why the symptoms are more prevalent in the evening. What we do know is that it is real, and needs to be recognized.

What can you do to help?

- Don't criticize negative feelings or poor judgment
- Encourage morning activities
- Provide for an afternoon nap
- Avoid arguments. Comfort, rather than scold
- Play quiet, relaxing music
- Limit number of evening visitors
- Avoid caffeine in the evening.
- Ask their Doctor about effects of medications
- Go for a late afternoon walk
- Show family videos or photographs
- Make failure-free activities readily available when they are looking for something to do
- Nurturing a well-behaved baby can be a relaxing activity
- Showing pictures of dolls or children can bring a smile or a positive reaction

Sundowning, in my opinion, is one of the symptoms of Alzheimer's disease that is often misunderstood, and can contribute to the difficulty of coping with other symptoms effectively.

What we do to relieve the symptoms with one person may increase the irritation of another. There is no clear answer that works for everyone. It is important to be aware of the signs, and have a variety of options to address those symptoms.

Helping Hints

- Close the drapes in the evening
- Keep lights on
- Keep music low
- Reduce demands
- Rocking in a chair
- Observe body language
- A warm bath can be relaxing
- Try leaving the TV on
- A massage is relaxing to some
- Warm milk is calming to others

It is usually more effective to schedule activities in the morning. For most residents, late afternoon is a good time to relax. Provide a variety of relaxing things to do, including soft music, a walk, reading, rocking, watching a favorite show, snack etc. Energetic evening activities can be non-productive for many residents.

I believe, as the loss of control and power becomes more apparent, fear, anxiety, frustration, paranoia and all Sundowners symptoms are likely to increase. In the evening, most residents are inactive, and have time to think about the light at the end of tunnel of life becoming dimmer. The help we can give them will brighten the light in their day and make the journey as pleasant as possible.

Hopefully, as a result of reading this chapter, you've discovered ways to reduce stress levels and improve willingness to participate in therapeutic activities. The next chapter will describe unique activities designed to further improve the quality of life for Alzheimer's sufferers.

Amira C. Tame, A.C.C.

Chapter 6

Custom Design an
Effective Activities Program

I had a resident who would only answer with "I don't know, yes, or no" over and over. Her family was frustrated because she communicated so little. They all assured me that she always loved children. I took several doll collector and nature magazines to her. I didn't ask her to say anything about the pictures, but I began making my own remarks. "I like this picture. This is such a pretty doll. This is not one of my favorites." During the first three sessions, she just sat, listened, and said little. During our fourth meeting, however, she said she had seen these magazines before, and began making comments like "Look how pretty this is." "This blue is a beautiful color." "This is so nice." "I like animals." She began to talk and communicate with gestures and emotional expressions. I was very pleased with the success of this approach.

Amira C. Tame, A.C.C.

No one said it would be easy

People with Alzheimer's are people to be loved. They are our mothers and fathers, our grandmothers and grandfathers.

One of the biggest challenges in providing care for a person with Alzheimer's is witnessing the mental decline and changes in personality and behavior. As the family member with Alzheimer's disease declines mentally, losses in function and awareness are often disturbing and difficult to handle. Be patient and understanding of how difficult it is for you.

For a close family member who is the primary caregiver, nothing hits harder than discovering you are no longer recognized by someone you care so much about. It feels as if the library has closed and your key doesn't open the door any more.

Activities are designed to stimulate memory function, improve quality of life, provide opportunities to share remaining memories, and keep the door open as long as possible. Your rewards come from seeing the positive results of your efforts.

There is no greater gift you can give a suffering person than relief and hope. Your relationship with your loved one will improve as you stimulate their positive memories and see self-confidence, physical and mental abilities improve.

Activities can be designed to accommodate any level of cognitive function or physical ability. In this chapter you will find a variety of flexible activities that will lay the groundwork for exciting techniques to improve the quality of life for the person with Alzheimer's.

If you have followed the guidelines in earlier chapters, you may already have seen a positive change in mood and attitude. You may also be seeing an improvement in your relationship with the person you're caring for. Removing obstacles from everyday life situations builds hope and trust that you can help them feel better.

The activities in this chapter are designed to provide mental and physical stimulation at any level of Alzheimer's disease. Activities that utilize the person's natural ability or ones that reflect past experiences can stimulate participation. Accenting the positive and de-emphasizing the negative will instill confidence and reduce their fear of failure.

Remember, participation is the key to success, not how well they do. Emphasize the importance of trying. Furthermore, maintaining a positive attitude about their condition and willingness to participate is essential. Your positive attitude is the greatest motivator and emotional healer available. A person with Alzheimer's who is having difficulty communicating will be influenced more by your body language (including eye contact, facial expressions, tonal voice, body movements) than any written or spoken attempts to communicate.

Positive changes in the person you're caring for will foster a positive attitude. Eventually, activities that were difficult become easier. Activities that were not possible prior to using these methods become possible. Understandably, it takes more time to learn new things for a person with Alzheimer's than it once did. Be patient and tolerant of the difficulties you encounter. Eventually, mood swings will be less frequent, and you will see a positive trend in overall mood. Don't press for intensive activities during a low time. Relaxing conversation or a special favorite activity might be most productive. Activities that produce **SPONTANEOUS** reactions are often useful when there is no interest in other activities. For times when no activities seem to produce a response, **PASSIVE** activities may be stimulating. If all else fails, you may have to resort to your list of **RESCUE** activities.

Important Guidelines

Medical Conditions

Be aware of any special medical conditions that might require medication or emergency treatment, such as:

1) Heart condition—Be sure to know where medication is located.
2) Seizures—Be aware of potential for seizures. How long do they last? How severe are they? What should you do if one occurs while the person is in your care? What medication should be taken?

3) Allergies—Know what allergies the person has and what symptoms to look for. An enjoyable walk in the woods or an outing to pick wildflowers could result in a very disappointing experience if the person is allergic to grass and trees, or reacts to pollen.

4) Food restrictions—The person you are caring for may have a diabetic condition that requires a strict diet. Any snack or treat could result in an acute reaction with serious consequences. Before offering any treats, gum, ice cream or fruits, determine what they can safely have.

These are only a few of the many possible medical conditions or restrictions you may need to be aware of. Prepare instructions, including a list of restrictions and medications, so anyone taking care of your loved one knows what to expect and what to do if an urgent situation occurs. Wearing an ID tag with name, address, blood type and acute medical conditions can speed emergency care and safe return if they wander away and get lost.

If you take the person with Alzheimer's out of the home, make sure you have all medications with you and know where the nearest emergency facility is located. Keep a list of any medical conditions and medications for that day. Information in the Personal Profile Form will be helpful. Keep a list of emergency phone numbers with you. The list should include the person designated to be notified in case of an emergency.

Minimize Injury Risks

The following precautions will minimize the risk of injury during activities:

Outside the facility

1) Obtain written authorization from the primary care facility or primary caregiver before leaving the facility for an off-site activity. Describe where you will be going and when you will return.

2) When you plan to take someone for a walk, consider their physical limitations when determining how far to go to make sure they will have enough energy to return. Make sure you will not be walking where they can wander into traffic or other areas where there is

an increased risk of injury (uneven sidewalks, grassy areas with holes, steep upgrades or downgrades, steps, loose gravel, etc.)

3) If you travel by car, a good policy is to not travel far from the care facility. If possible, travel toward a health care facility, rather than away from one. A cell phone can save time if you have to call 911 or other emergency numbers. Knowing first aid techniques will help you when an emergency situation arises.

Items used during activities

1) Small marbles or pieces of colored parts can be mistaken for candy and could cause injury. Avoid using such items in later stage Alzheimer's or be very attentive while engaging in activities that include small parts. Do not use any items with sharp edges.

2) Make sure activity items or other heavy items are not stored or placed on a high shelf or cabinet. These items could fall and cause injuries.

3) Use plastic or dull knives to cut vegetables and fruits.

4) Never use glass items that could break if dropped.

5) Always provide close supervision when you are near fire or heat (baking, stove top-cooking, outside barbecues, campfires). Make sure hot items are out of reach. Ensure that paper products, cloth or clothing do not come in contact with the fire or hot surface.

What Is An Activity?

Activity, as defined by the American Heritage Dictionary, is "any energetic action or movement, a specified form of supervised action."

For a person with Alzheimer's, activities do not have to be physical or energetic. Therapeutic activities can stimulate physical or mental activity or a combination of both. Physically stimulating activities can be either organized exercises or spontaneous reactions to a stimulus initiated by the caregiver. Mental exercises programmed to the individual's abilities can be very motivating and rewarding for both the client and the caregiver. Some of the activities do not require direct supervision. An example is squeezing a soft ball for finger and hand exercises that also provides relief for frustrations and anxiety, without being supervised by the caregiver. Alzheimer's disease has created a clear need for therapeutic activities, which in turn have redefined the meaning of and benefit of activities as we've known them.

Types of Activities

Activities are defined by participation, stimulus, purpose and rescue.

Participation

Active

Active participation **requires an action** by the participant. Any oral response or motor gesture constitutes active participation. Any response, whether spoken, written or physical, is considered active participation. Examples of active participation are: conversing, game playing, arts and crafts, walking, singing, dressing, writing a letter, exercising, gardening etc.

Passive

Passive participation **does not require interaction** between the person with Alzheimer's and the caregiver. A passive activity only requires willingness to participate. No physical or emotional response is required. Passive activities are the most basic form of activity and, by utilizing proper techniques, could lead to active participation.

Listening to music or conversations, watching television or live entertainment, watching the caregiver or others performing activities such as cooking, cleaning, dancing, and exercising are passive activities that can stimulate active participation. Getting a beauty treatment or massage can be very relaxing and improve willingness to participate in other activities.

Focus

Activities designed for **mental stimulation** may include some physical activity, but the primary focus is to improve memory function.

Mental stimulation may result in an oral response, a judgment, or a decision. Mentally-focused activities include reading aloud, spelling, object recognition, recall questions, picture recognition, singing, sights and sound, etc. Examples of mentally-focused activities that require physical participation are: card games, Dominoes, picture puzzles, mail box, stacking cups, sorting items and treasure hunt.

Activities focused on **physical improvement** can include mental stimulation, but the primary focus is to improve physical dexterity. Physical activities require the use of motor skills to participate. Generally, any physical activity performed at any level will be beneficial. Some motor skills degrade because they believe a hand, arm, or leg doesn't work anymore. Often a spontaneous physical response can jog memory and results in restoring a diminished motor skill. Examples of activities that stimulate motor skills are: physical exercises, walking, riding an adult tricycle, squeezing a ball, balloon toss, putting a golf ball, and unwinding twine. Many physical activities can improve strength and coordination and reconnect mental awareness to physical ability. Examples of physical activities that also invoke mental stimulation are knitting, crocheting, sewing, crafts, painting, gardening, basket weaving, and model building.

Stimulus

Stimulation techniques can affect the outcome of any activity session. Activities can be either **spontaneous** or **organized**. Many activities start out as planned and organized and with repetition become spontaneous. Be flexible when things don't go as planned. Use your repertoire of skills to find something that does work. You may venture through many spontaneous reactions before finding an organized activity that works. Many times, spontaneous activities are all you engage in at one session. Usually spontaneous sessions allow some self expression and control in the direction the session is taking. Spontaneous activities need only be controlled to the extent they are not destructive or in total chaos. Spontaneous activities include playing catch with a soft ball, bumping a balloon back and forth, kicking a soft ball on the floor. Examples of organized activities are: card games, spelling games, Bingo, word scramble games, exercise routines. Most organized activities have rules, or a routine to follow, and are much easier to manage if the person is capable or in the mood.

Purpose

Functional activities are designed to improve one's ability to perform day-to-day tasks. Improvement can usually be realized in the areas of hygiene, eating, dressing, grooming, cleaning, organizing laundry, etc. Functional activities include cooking together, preparing cut vegetables, cleaning their room, vacuuming, washing and putting away dishes. Walk to rooms with them so they become familiar with the route. Utensils used for functional activities can be used in other activities to keep them familiar with what they are used for. Motor/oral skills and social interaction can improve as functional activities reduce stress, anxiety and fear of failure.

Entertaining activities provide a break from the routine of working on skill improvement. They are designed to provide a relaxing and enjoyable time. Surprising results can be achieved by not focusing on any skill improvement. Examples include a trip to the airport to watch airplanes (memories of flying may stimulate conversation), watching a favorite movie, listening to favorite music, or going to a shopping mall.

Rescue

Rescue activities are those you know are **most effective** in situations where there is no interest in activities or there are overwhelming barriers that obstruct participation in activities. Keep a list of activities that have always worked at some level. They may be as simple as going for an ice cream, chewing gum, or just sharing quiet time. Sometimes a foot or hand massage will relax the person and be conducive to conversation, or provide a conduit to participation in another activity.

How to be Successful at Any Ability Level

Although Alzheimer's is a progressively degenerating disease, often the symptoms can be curtailed or slowed resulting in marked behavioral improvements. Anyone with Alzheimer's can participate in activities at some level. Games can be broken down into progressive levels even within the same activity. As an example, a person in the early stage of Alzheimer's can participate actively in more complicated activities such as card games. As the disease progresses, it becomes more difficult to remember how to play and to focus long enough to finish a game. As activities become more difficult they can be adjusted to declining abilities.

A person in the advanced stage of Alzheimer's with low mental function can handle only very simple tasks, and a card game may consist of recognizing numbers, suits, or colors, red or black cards or just turning the cards over and stacking them. You can always design an activity for which the person is capable of participating.

Cards are only one example of how activities can be broken down to their simplest form. All activities can be customized to suit the participant's specific abilities and interests. Design each activity so the participant can be successful. Remember, they don't have to do things right to be successful. They only need to feel good about what they've done.

Encourage participation of a resistant person by involving them with passive activities such as listening to music, singing, watching you or others perform an activity, eating a snack or chewing gum.

Focus on Available Senses

If the resident has a history of mental impairment, it may be difficult to draw upon past experiences to develop activities. Activities will require creative and flexible techniques that are customized during each session. Interest in activities may fluctuate from one extreme to another at any level. Make the best use of the available emotional up swings and expect less during the down time.

Usually you can detect productive opportunities and overcome most communication obstacles, regardless of the mental or physical challenges they might have. You must work within their abilities. The person may have experienced some functional or sensory loss prior to the onset of Alzheimer's disease that they have already learned to cope with. Know these limitations before beginning an activities session.

Diminished Sight

Finding out that their eyesight is too poor to read after you give them a good book to read is too late. If diminishing sight has been a problem for many years, it is possible that other senses have been enhanced to compensate for the loss of vision. Use the senses that remain functional in your activities.

The treasure hunt game is an example of one activity that doesn't require good eyesight. Items can be identified by touch and feel. Recognizing various articles without sight can restore self-confidence. You may be surprised at how rewarding this activity can be.

Sense of Smell

Aroma therapy is a useful activity that compensates for the loss of sight and may stimulate memories associated with the aroma. Sense of smell is often enhanced as other senses are diminished. Taking walks past flower gardens, smelling fruits and vegetables, and using touch and smell activities and scented candles can provide a variety of smells that may be familiar. You do not have to light the candle to smell the aroma. Coffee grounds also have a distinct aroma that is familiar to most people and can often be recognized. If the person has no idea what the aroma is, you can give a hint by asking if it smells like coffee. When the person describes a smell that doesn't match the object, don't correct their answer. What smells like one thing to one may smell like something else to another.

Sounds Good to Them

Sounds are effective for stimulating memory and conversation. Hearing sounds of jets leaving, announcements on the PA system, and people talking about their trips can stimulate memories of places they've traveled to. For those who are not able to make a trip to the airport, just listening to recorded sounds of airport activity can be stimulating. Sounds of train whistles or traffic can also stimulate memories of trips. Sounds of nature can be relaxing for some. Sounds of birds singing, doves cooing, crickets chirping, water flowing in a stream, etc. may stimulate fond memories.

Therapeutic Activities

Hopefully, you now realize the benefit of preparing therapeutic activities. Quality time can now be focused on activities that help improve quality of life, physical/mental health, and memory capacity. With these changes come improved attitudes, higher self-esteem and restored relationships.

These guidelines will will be your roadmap to success

1) Before selecting any activity, determine whether the person lacks, or is deficient in, any motor skills or sensory functions.
2) Select a previously familiar activity.
3) Select a level of difficulty that matches the available abilities.
4) Gradually increase the level of difficulty as you see improvement.
5) Give recognition and rewards for participation and progress.
6) Provide feedback to family members so the progress is recognized.
7) Monitor the improvements and document the progress periodically to keep track of which activities are most effective (Activities Progress Report in Chapter 3).

Communication

How many times have you heard that effective communication is critical to success ? It is no different with Alzheimer's. Improved communication can trigger memories and lead to greater self confidence, more trust, less anger, and can open the door to participation with activities.

Conversation Stimulation

When your loved one is unable to talk or cannot think of anything to say because of difficulty forming sentences, show magazines with pictures of topics associated with hobbies or other subjects that were important in their past (animals, babies, flowers, faces, etc.). Ask what are in the pictures and which things are liked most. Mention things that you like in the pictures to help break the ice. Their response can help determine the direction of the conversation. Don't force the conversation in a direction you may want it to go. Open your conversations by talking about simple things. Make it as easy as possible for them to respond to your questions. Start with questions with yes/no answers. Do you like this color, do you like this car, house, furniture etc. are all non-threatening questions with no wrong answers. Allowing the conversation to flow with the person's interest will help them feel in control without excessive pressure. Your questions provide stimulation to recall thoughts, feelings and events and demonstrate a genuine interest in the special care you are providing.

Giving key words or details about an event or activity can stimulate memory. One woman could not recall visiting a particular garage sale until she was reminded of the special antique she had found there. She had a strong emotional connection to the antique that triggered memory of the outing. Key words/subjects could include: childhood, area where they grew up, first date or love; friends, teachers, proms, graduation, girlfriends, jobs, education, military service.

Take advantage of recall opportunities whenever possible. As an example, one man triggered many memories when he said, "I remember a Mardi Gras celebration." I told him it sounded exciting and I would love to hear more. If you show empathy and interest, your sincerity will be apparent, and with time more memories will be forthcoming. Always listen closely to anything being shared by a person with Alzheimer's. Their stories need to be told.

Write a letter to a family member

Writing letters has many benefits. Many persons with Alzheimer's have lost confidence in their ability to communicate well. It is not important that the words make perfect sense or the letter is only a few words long. The process of writing and your willingness to help is important. If there is nothing to write about, suggest writing a statement about how they feel.

Often, they will feel very close to you after writing down their feelings. The letter does not have to be sent to the person they are writing to. The real benefit comes from communicating thoughts and feelings through writing.

Reminiscing

Reminiscing about positive experiences you've had with your loved one will not only help heal the wounds of Alzheimer's disease, but will also help heal the wounds you've been feeling as a result of the disease.

Reminisce about school days

Know beforehand which grade level was completed. Some are capable of recalling their college years or graduate school, while others did not complete grade school. (This information is in the Personal Profile Form.) Usually there are many memories associated with education. If they attended college or graduate school, it may be where friendship led to marriage. They would have many memories to talk about. Most people like to hear how smart you think they are, regardless of education level. Some like to brag about how much they accomplished in life with minimal education.

Reminisce about important people/places

Reminiscing about former presidents, other world leaders, famous actors or significant historical events, usually results in emotional recollections. Former union members may want to discuss union activities related to work experience. Retired longtime employees of one company may recall a former boss or close co-workers. Famous people who have made history, such as artists, inventors, mathematicians, or great athletes may be recalled.

Discussing celebrities or famous people (actors, politicians, singers, musicians) from the early years of the person's life can help stimulate thoughts of respected people. It is sometimes easier to recall details or contributions of a famous person's life than aspects of one's own. It is possible that certain celebrities were significant role models. Just as major events in one's life are easier to recall, so is a celebrity who identifies with the "good old days."

Romantic recollections

Romantic experiences in younger days are usually remembered as good times. Don't be specific when asking about earlier relationships. It is important to be general about early romances.

There may have been some difficult situations (alcohol abuse, physical abuse) that one may not want to talk about. Let them decide which relationship they are willing to talk about. Sometimes romantic times, that are filled with emotions, are more easily recalled than other memories.

Listen to music/songs

Some favorite songs are listed in the Personal Profile Form (Chapter 3) under likes and dislikes. If it looks like you truly enjoy these songs too, it might stimulate memories of good times when they sang with family members. This activity may stimulate a story or two that can be shared. If you don't get a response while listening, try humming the tune softly and see if there is interest in joining in.

- If the person has a strong religious background, try songs with a religious theme that can be sung or played to lift their spirits and help recall past holidays. Carry the good cheer generated from these sessions for as long as possible. Throughout the session, reflect on the joy you feel listening to the uplifting songs.
- Listening to old songs is a great way to stimulate thoughts about earlier times and past experiences. They may recall a particular song from the past and recall the year when it was popular. Old camp songs are often remembered. Singers like Kate Smith, Bing Crosby, and Frank Sinatra are a few of the all-time favorites from the past.
- Songs associated with seasons can trigger memories of holidays or other seasonal events. Some examples are: "White Christmas," "April Showers," "Summertime," "You Are My Sunshine," "Autumn Leaves," "April in Paris," and "Singing in the Rain."
- Songs associated with cities, states or places can bring back memories of favorite places or events. Examples include: "The Yellow Rose of Texas," "North to Alaska," "I Left My Heart in San Francisco," "Tennessee Waltz," "My Old Kentucky Home," "New York," and "By the Time I Get to Phoenix."
- Songs associated with people or names can stimulate memories of acquaintances or special relationships. Examples are: "Goodnight Irene," "Danny Boy," and "Rambling Rose."
- Love songs can often stimulate emotional recollections. Some examples of love songs are: "Love is a Many Splendored Thing," "Somewhere My Love," Because of You," and "Let Me Call You Sweetheart."

Look at family photographs

Family photographs are often helpful in building pride and self-confidence. Looking at photos of family members may trigger memories of loving experiences they had. Photos are reminders of the many responsibilities they've had and can generate recollections about child rearing.

It is not important to recall each person's name or face in the photos. Looking through the photos is the important aspect of this activity. It is OK if the person can't recall the names of people in the photos. There is no significance in correcting them. Children's pictures often bring smiles and positive comments. Viewing the photos without expecting correct recollection of details or faces will help reduce anxiety and encourage conversation.

Family photo albums can be kept near so they are easy to find. Often, persons with Alzheimer's want to sit quietly looking at their personal possessions, opening and closing drawers and checking things out. I often see them sitting quietly and flipping through the pages of familiar photo albums.

Make a family tree poster

This can be created with information from the Personal Profile Form (Chapter 3), or by talking to other caregivers. The closest family members should be included. If there is a picture or name that irritates the person you are caring for, consider removing that information. Eventually, you may be able to resolve the irritation and restore the missing information. This is not a legal family tree and is being done only for the purpose of stimulating conversation with family members.

Look up familiar names in the Yellow Pages or business directory

This helps them recall memories of stores where they used to shop. Choose well-known stores or speciality stores they've shopped in. This activity is thought provoking and helps focus attention on positive recollections. Going through an alphabetical list of names encourages organized thinking. Looking up store names can generate many opportunities to recall enjoyable memories about special purchases at a particular store.

Amira C. Tame, A.C.C.

Reminisce about a favorite season

This activity encourages recall of happy days in a particular season and will, hopefully, stimulate positive thoughts to lighten the person's mood. Vacations, trips, friends, and family members are all part of the person's memories of past activities (e.g., boating, skiing, walks, picnics). After they share seasonal favorites with you, share some of your own memorable experiences from the same season. Asking about memories of activities or events that occurred during specific seasons narrows the scope, making it easier to remember the events.

Daily Functional

Clipping coupons

Sometimes sale items require cutting coupons out of a flyer or newspaper. This gives the person a renewed feeling of being frugal. Even if it is to help lower your shopping bill and not theirs, it may stimulate memories of past responsibilities and conversation about familiar shopping experiences. The cutting provides finger and hand exercises and promotes hand/eye coordination. Use scissors that are designed to be safe for children. They will not have a pointed end or sharp edges that could be harmful.

Cleaning up after meals

Often, a person with Alzheimer's will be able to recall mealtime activities. After finishing a meal or an activity in the kitchen, let them help clear items that are safe to handle and take them to the sink. If you wipe the table, let them dry it off with a clean towel. Let them wash and dry unbreakable dishes or perform other tasks they are capable of. This activity will give them a feeling of being useful and needed. Make sure all the dishware is unbreakable and utensils are not sharp.

Grooming

Manicuring—At times residents are not in the mood for activities. A manicure or some pampering (foot or hand massage) is generally much appreciated. Cutting toenails or fingernails is not only relaxing but a necessary grooming task. She may want to put on lipstick or makeup and may need your help. Make her feel good. Tell her she looks attractive. A massage may be relaxing enough to share feelings. Good hygiene and appearance always have a positive influence. If possible, groom in front of a mirror so the person can see the pampering and feel a part of what is taking place. Always use a hand lotion recommended by staff or family so you don't risk an allergic reaction.

Hand Washing—If possible, provide a familiar brand of soap, wash cloth, towel, sponge and soap dish. Using familiar soap will avoid allergic reactions. Hand washing should not be rushed. Washing hands with a gentle massaging action relaxes the fingers, hands and wrists. Make sure they wash their hands before meals and before leaving the bathroom. Memories of good hygiene will be reinforced through this simple activity.

Dressing techniques—Persons with Alzheimer's often have difficulty dressing because they forgot how to fasten their clothing. To help retrain them, use items of clothing, such as skirts, shirts, pants, blouses, that can be buttoned, zipped, snapped or hooked in activities. Select an item of clothing to button or unbutton, zip or unzip, hook or unhook. Start with only two items and gradually increase the selection pool. This activity will improve dexterity and memory and serve to enhance self-confidence when dressing.

Raking leaves

Raking leaves gives a sense of accomplishment and of being helpful. It renews feelings of pride and ownership, and is an opportunity to be outside of the home. Light raking, with your help, can provide exercise and the satisfaction of being able to help with a chore and improve the appearance of their home. Light raking without any lifting provides exercise without over exertion.

Vacuuming carpet

This activity promotes cleanliness and gives a sense of ownership and authority. It can reduce frustration and provide exercise without the person leaving their room. How well one cleans is not nearly as important as participation. If they are not able to plug the sweeper into the electrical outlet without being harmed, you plug it in.

Watering house plants

House plants provide color and beauty. Flowers can also be therapeutic because of their calming effect and their role in special occasions. Reminding them of the role plants play in producing oxygen will reinforce the need to keep them healthy.

Weeding the flower bed

Weeding is a familiar activity. They can feel pride and a sense of ownership in being able to help keep their home beautiful. Most people do not mind weeding periodically. This activity requires hand-eye coordination and is an excellent mental exercise. One must decide if a plant needs to stay or is a weed and should be pulled. Don't be critical if a wrong plant is pulled.

After repeated trips to the flower garden she might remember that a particular plant is one that should not be removed. Check the garden beforehand to make sure there are no dangerous plants in the garden (poison ivy or plants with prickers on stems, etc.). Encourage good posture and stay close at all times to ensure they're not eating the plants. Gloves are highly recommended because even nonpoisonous plants can cause an allergic reaction.

Folding clothes

Folding clothes can be a very stimulating activity for a person with Alzheimer's. Touching and feeling the fabrics brings back memories of when they folded clothes for their families. They may also recall how to fold certain items in certain ways. Additional stimuli can be gained by sorting socks by color, patterns, men's, women's, children's, etc. It's a good feeling to help with this chore, and end up with matching pairs of socks. If the person is not able to distinguish patterns and/or colors well, give them socks that have striking differences (bright colors or bold patterns) which can be easily sorted.

Folding towels

Folding towels is easier than folding clothes, so it is broken down into a separate activity. Persons with Alzheimer's usually find folding towels a fairly simple task because most towels have the same shape and require similar steps. It is also a relaxing activity that is not frustrating because it leaves little room for error. The activity can begin with a small wash cloth that will be easy to fold, and progress to larger bath towels which are more difficult. Eventually sheets and other bedding can be tackled. The key to success is the uniform shape of towels. Once you fold one, it is easier to fold the next.

Washing tableware

Tableware is easy to pick up and won't break if dropped. If the person you're caring for is afraid of dropping dishes, ask for help with the tableware instead. Always remove any sharp knives before asking for help. Because tableware is smaller, easier to handle, and unbreakable, the person won't be afraid of handling them. Don't be critical of water spots or tableware that is not as clean as you would like. You can re-wash the utensils later without the person knowing. Even though the dishes or tableware are not washed well, always show appreciation for their help. After cleaning, the person can put the tableware in a tray or organizer. Put at least one utensil in each slot to provide a pattern to follow. Sorting sizes and shapes is easy and stimulating at the same time. It provides a sense of helping with necessary chores. A common fear among persons with Alzheimer's is being a burden on others. You can greatly reduce their fear by giving them something to do that makes them feel useful and helpful to you.

Meal & Food Preparation

Baking

This is a very stimulating experience for a person with Alzheimer's, especially if they have baked in the past. Biscuits, dinner rolls and filled fruit pies are easily baked from ready-to-bake packages, or can be made from scratch.

A person may remember some or all the steps for preparing their favorite recipes. This activity provides ample opportunity to stimulate fond memories. If they have never baked before, they may have wanted to, but never got the chance. The aroma of baking cookies can be a strong reminder of enjoyable times and events associated with baking. If someone is assisting you in the preparation, pay close attention to every step of the activity to ensure a safe and successful outcome.

For those not able to measure ingredients, pre-measure them. The wide variety of pre-mixed cookie doughs available provides an opportunity to satisfy the sweet tooth of any person with a favorite cookie treat. Some cookie dough is already prepared. You only have to slice the dough and it is ready to bake. Allow them to do as much as possible. Preheat the oven to the proper temperature setting. Set a timer so you can do other activities without watching the clock. There is a fine line between being overbearing and giving them the comfort of knowing you are there to help and guide them. They need to feel that the activity is something they contributed to. By just watching and participating in little ways, persons can feel involved and experience a sense of self-accomplishment.

Baking homemade bread is an activity that provides good physical and mental stimulation. The physical part comes from preparing, kneading and rolling the dough. The mental part comes from measuring and combining all of the ingredients. If all of this is too difficult, ready-made dough can be purchased that still requires kneading, rolling and flouring. Participating in the baking process, enjoying the aroma, and tasting the rewards all provide motivation to complete the activity. Aroma of cooking can linger long after the activity has ended and continue to be stimulating and thought-provoking.

Making fruit juice

Orange juice, grapefruit juice and lemonade can be homemade. The fruit can be cut, squeezed and mixed with water, providing a feeling of accomplishment because the drink was prepared from scratch.

Often, preparing things from scratch (as they used to do)gives a feeling of power generated from knowing they can do something on their own and is a great esteem booster. If you are concerned about letting someone use a knife because they may cut themselve, cut the fruit yourself or provide a plastic knife that will still cut the fruit but greatly reduces the chance of injury. If it is too risky to use a knife at all, bring pre-cut fruit that only requires squeezing and mixing with water.

Making a stove-top pie

This is made with two pieces of bread and any filling (e.g., applesauce, jelly, canned pie fillings, or pizza ingredients). Using a clam-like cooker (such as a trail pie maker used mainly with campfires), place the filled slices of bread in one of the halves and close the cooker. The long handles usually include a hook to keep them shut tightly. Remove any of the bread pieces that extend outside the pie maker mold. Then hold each side over the stove for a few minutes. The result is an almost instantaneous, successful stove-top pie. It requires little assistance or preparation in advance by the caregiver. Few ingredients, and a little patience can result in a tasty, enjoyable treat.

Instead. Always remove any sharp knives before asking for help. Because tableware is smaller, easier to handle, and unbreakable, the person won't be afraid of handling them. Don't be critical of water spots or tableware that is not as clean as you would like. You can re-wash the utensils later without the person knowing. Even though the dishes or tableware are not washed well, always show appreciation for their help. After cleaning, the person can put the tableware in a tray or organizer. Put at least one utensil in each slot to provide a pattern to follow. Sorting sizes and shapes is easy and stimulating at the same time. It provides a sense of helping with necessary chores. A common fear among persons with Alzheimer's is being a burden on others. You can greatly reduce their fear by giving them something to do that makes them feel useful and helpful to you.

NOTE: Caution must be taken with this activity as the metal part of the handles get hot. Also, if the extra bread around the cooker is not removed before cooking, it may catch on fire.

Making coffee

Making coffee from scratch can be fun. With so many prepared foods and automated processes available today, it's fun sometimes to step back and do things the old way. Start your session with a drive to a local coffee

Amira C. Tame, A.C.C.

shop where fresh-roasted coffee beans are available. Let the person select a favorite flavor and have the sales associate roast and grind the beans. Select a dessert to share when the coffee is ready. The atmosphere in most coffee shops is easygoing and comfortable. The person most likely will enjoy this activity because it is reminder of the days when making coffee from fresh, ground beans was more common.

Back at home, if they are able to help, ask them to measure appropriate quantities of water and coffee to put in the coffee pot. You can both enjoy a fresh cup of coffee and dessert.

Having afternoon tea or coffee

It is sometimes beneficial to have a simple social affair. It need not always be a mental or physical activity, but simply a sharing time together. Having a relaxing warm drink can create an atmosphere for opening up and sharing whatever thoughts come to mind. If a light snack is available, feel free to share something appropriate. Hot cider is a drink that may bring back memories of a cider mill trip, or when cider was made at home.

Barbecuing outside

An outside barbecue can bring back fond memories of favorite foods, family members, and picnics associated with family gatherings and holidays. If a grill is available, many foods can be barbecued outside (potatoes, meat, hot dogs, vegetables). It speeds up the process if food that requires a long time to cook is precooked and only needs warming. Foods can also be wrapped in foil to make it easier and less messy. Be careful to light the barbecue before anyone comes close to it and supervise actions at all times.

Popping corn

This is a popular snack food that can be easily prepared. Listening to the corn pop and enjoying the aroma provide sensory effects that may stimulate thoughts about past sports events, movies, and family get-togethers. If you are concerned that someone might choke on the popcorn or be harmed in any way, mention that you need their assistance in preparing the popcorn for a function later that day. They will enjoy knowing they made something for a worthwhile purpose.

Making a fruit salad

This activity is fun and produces a healthy, tasty treat. Many fruits can be used. Some fruits provide many opportunities for the person to participate. Bananas can be peeled and/or sliced, apples can be peeled and/or sliced and strawberries/cherries can be washed and cut. Encourage them to do as much as possible independently. If you see them struggling, offer assistance. For safety, provide plastic knives for cutting fruits and vegetables. As each fruit is prepared, the aroma becomes stronger and more enjoyable. If the person handpicked certain fruits as a youngster or liked to have certain fruits in cereal, fruit can provide many opportunities for conversation. Eating the salad can stimulate recollection of dinners with loved ones. Visitors might enjoy a snack they prepared for them.

Making sandwiches

This is a stimulating activity because a sandwich is simple to prepare, easy to clean up and is a tasty treat. Preparing this snack may stimulate memories of the many lunches or picnics made in the past for children, spouses or grandchildren. If a favorite snack sandwich is not in the Personal Profile Form (Chapter 3), you can substitute any easy-to-prepare sandwiches. Begin the activity by asking where the ingredients and utensils are to make the sandwiches. They can help by putting bread on the table and assist in preparing the sandwiches.

Making a birthday cake

Check the completed survey form that notes special days in the person's life. It is highly recommended that you always celebrate a person's birthday in some way. Try to make the person feel very special. The Personal Profile Form indicates preferred types of cakes. If possible, bake a cake with the person and allow them time to decorate the cake. Even if their birthday was not celebrated in the past, they will still enjoy and appreciate your effort in making their birthday a special day. If they can't help much with the preparation, they will still feel honored that you are celebrating their birthday. Most enjoy decorating their room as part of the celebration.

Shelling nuts

Most in early stage Alzheimer's can do this. Pistachios, for example, can be opened without a nutcracker and provide finger exercise. Ask if they recall when pistachios were colored red and it was difficult to find uncolored ones. They may recall eating pistachios and ending up with red-stained lips and fingers. If you see that they are having difficulty opening the nuts, have a nutcracker handy for assistance. With more alert persons, a variety of nuts can be cracked, chopped and prepared for a snack or fruit salad.

The following are examples of exercise-focused activities.

Exercise

Exercise For Your Body and Brain

Consider the following benefits of exercise for your loved one:

- Improves sleep—Taking a walk during the day may expend enough energy so they become ready for a restful sleep at night.
- Improves appetite—Exercising works up a healthy appetite. Your loved one may eat a better meal if they have been physically active.
- Reduces agitation and wandering—Physical activity could help divert attention and reduce the likelihood of wandering.

The risk for developing Alzheimer's disease can be reduced by reading books or magazines, walking, watching movies or visiting friends or relatives. Reading and engaging in other leisure activities may reduce the risk or delay onset of clinical manifestations of dementia, according to a new study published in Neurology, the scientific journal of the American Academy of Neurology. High education and occupational attainments have previously been associated with reduced risk of Alzheimer's. This study demonstrates the benefits of leisure activities in reducing the risk of dementia among people of any education or occupation. "Our study suggests that aspects of life experience supply a set of skills or repertoires that allow an individual to cope with progressing Alzheimer's Disease pathology for a longer time before the disease becomes clinically apparent," said Stern. "Maintaining intellectual and social engagement through participation in everyday activities seems to buffer healthy individuals against cognitive decline in later life."

Hula Hoop

Yes!! Even a person with Alzheimer's can enjoy exercising with a hula hoop. Of course, they must be supervised and guided to use it in a safe way and at their individual skill level. It is easier to do this exercise activity while sitting in a chair with arms. It helps make them more secure, and provides a place to grip and help them balance. Hold the hoop with outstretched arms as you would a steering wheel of a car. Rotate the hoop left and right without releasing the hoop, as if you are changing lanes in a car. You can start with hands held close together and gradually move them as far apart as possible. Now, rotate the hoop as if you are making a full left turn by swapping your grip from left to right as you rotate the hoop.

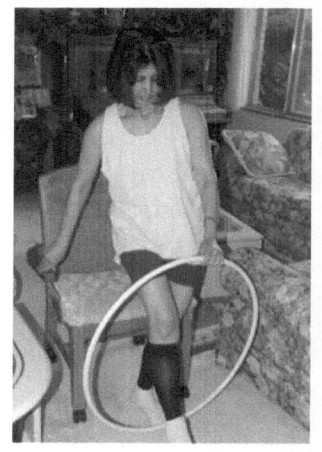

Reverse the direction you are rotating and make several more full right turn revolutions. Still sitting in a chair, and holding the hoop with both hands, place the hoop over your head until it touches the chair, and rotate the hoop back over your head until it touches the floor. Do this several times before moving on to the next exercise. While they are still sitting, and the hoop is rotated to the floor, ask them to put one foot through the hoop and touch the floor, and bring it back through and touch the floor again. Do this several times. Repeat this with the other foot, and then with both feet at the same time. If they are able to, while the hoop is rotated to the floor, ask them to stand up and step through the hoop and bring it up over their head as they sit back down.

This can also be done in reverse. Stand close to them so you can help them keep their balance. They can hold onto the chair arm with one hand while they are stepping through the hoop. It will help support them. Another good exercise is for them to roll the hoop on the floor as they walk. This encourages walking while stimulating hand/eye coordination.

Taking a walk

Take a walk around the facility in a safe area where you can sit and talk. Sometimes, walks are simply moving from one chair to another. Persons with Alzheimer's usually do not try to leave the area if you are close by. A walk generally relieves anger and frustration and, at the same time, provides fresh air. After returning indoors, continue with therapy activities so they don't connect going back indoors with your visit being over.

When you walk with a person with Alzheimer's, walk at a pace that is not over exerting for either of you. Offer support when needed. Take time to see all the sights around you, making comments about the fragrance of the flowers, animals you see, and whatever trees you may see. Ask what the person's favorites are. Giving individual attention will usually result in their sharing thoughts with you and build on the trusting relationship. Often a person with Alzheimer's will want to return home quickly while out for a walk. Encourage longer walks by suggesting alternate routes to the same destination. Suggesting a walk to the lounge or snack area might provide an incentive to participate.

Playing catch

This helps improve hand/eye coordination, encourages reflex responses, is stimulating and fun. You can roll a soft ball back and forth or ask her to kick it back to strengthen leg muscles. Work with her to control how far or how hard the ball is rolled or thrown. Let her know if it is returned too hard or in the wrong direction. Spontaneous reactions are sometimes the first indication that she is ready to participate.

A balloon does not follow the same trajectery each time you strike it, so spontaneous reactions and focused attention are elements of this activity. When a balloon is tossed to a person, the natural and spontaneous reaction is to bump it back. This will encourage people to use their hands and arms in a way that provides exercise for their upper body muscles.

Soft Ball & Balloon Toss

Many soft ball exercises can be very relaxing at any stage of dementia. Sponge balls can be used to play catch, roll across a table, or kick back and forth on the floor, without fear of injury. Squeezing a soft ball, or tossing a balloon is a simple, relaxing hand exercise that can help reduce stress and frustrations.

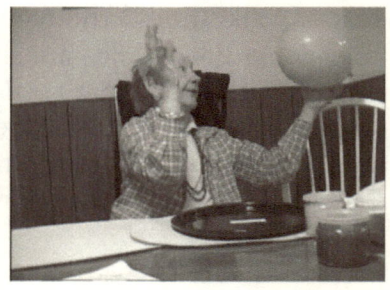

Tossing a balloon to the player will trigger spontaneous reactions such as hitting it back, or trying to catch the balloon.

Molding with play dough

This is an excellent activity because kneading the dough provides exercise for fingers. They can create whatever forms they like with the dough, or simply roll it around in free form shapes. Emphasize that the dough is being used for exercise purposes and is good for both hands and fingers. Let the person know that adults use clay for artwork and also for models of automobiles to see what they look like before the actual car is made.

Squeezing a soft ball

Squeezing a ball is a good hand exercise that can relax a person with Alzheimer's, encourage spontaneous gestures, and can be done without supervision. If you explain the benefit of strengthening fingers and hand muscles, most will be happy to participate. To stimulate interest, start squeezing the ball yourself to show how easy and safe it is. You may have to explain the benefit of strong fingers and hands for some to participate. This may be a group activity, and may encourage social interaction.

Lifting exercises for arms and wrists

A gallon jug can be used to provide a means of progressively increasing weight by filling it with water as muscles strengthen. The handle on the container provides a convenient way to grasp the jug.

Leg exercises

The most common and useful leg exercise is walking. It provides an opportunity to socialize and offers a change of environment. Other exercises can be done while sitting in a chair. Lifting one leg at a time and bending the knee will improve upper and lower leg strength. Kicking a soft ball or balloon is also a low-impact leg exercise.

Weaving a basket

It is easy to complete a basket from a partially woven plastic basket. Choose a basket with bright, contrasting colors so you can follow the original pattern. If the person is capable of weaving the basket without your help, have one for each of you so they can observe your methods. If not, you can work on one basket together. The hand/eye coordination and physical hand/finger exercises and mental stimulation provide an opportunity for a very satisfying activity.

Finishing simple rhyming songs

Begin a familiar old-time rhyme with the first verse and see if the person can complete the next. Songs can be of the person's choosing or ones familiar to you. Sometimes the person can teach you one they still recall. Folk songs such as "She'll Be Coming 'Round the Mountain," "You Are My Sunshine," or "On Top of Old Smoky" are usually good choices.

Verbal Activities

Reading aloud (short stories about favorite subjects)

This is a beneficial activity, especially if the person with Alzheimer's can read without help or with minimal assistance from you. Putting together thoughts in words through reading allows them to visualize and vocalize words they may not have seen or spoken for many years. Repeated reading may bring back memories of reading in school or reading to children. If the person can't read, reading to them may stimulate thoughts (friends, families, experiences) by hearing stories from years past. Listening to stories can be a relaxing experience, especially if the stories are about subjects the person has some recollection of.

Reader's Digest is recommended because it offers a variety of reading material (short stories, jokes, anecdotes) and is available in large print. It is also an older publication that many persons may remember from childhood or young adult years. Words that the person previously did not recognize are often recognized when associated with familiar text and pictures.

Reading the daily newspaper

This gives the person you're caring for a chance to enjoy something they may have liked to do in their past. It is important to remove the sensitive sections of the newspaper beforehand (especially local crimes and obituaries). Reading the newspaper is a way to keep abreast of what's happening in the world, and may be important to them. Even if they don't understand all the details, reading about current events can help them feel they are a part of society. It also provides other fun opportunities, such as crossword or wordsearch puzzles, trivia games, finding a favorite section, searching for various pictures or words throughout the paper, etc. Leave the newspaper with the person when you leave, because it could stimulate interest later.

Asking simple trivia questions

Answering trivia questions correctly about the "old days" can help elevate a person's self-esteem. Answers do not have to be exactly right, and you can say you are not sure of the answers either, so no one will feel intimidated by what you know. If the person is in the early stages of Alzheimer's disease, the questions could be more complex. Regardless, the questions should be associated with familiar subjects. If the Personal Profile Form indicates that golf was a hobby, then golf trivia questions would be appropriate. If the person liked sports in general, then the questions could be broader in scope. The more you know about the person's interests, the better you can formulate questions that will be correctly answered.

Unwinding ribbon or twine

Tightly wrapped, colored, plastic ribbon or twine can be used to decorate various projects after being unwound. Unwinding twine is a great finger exercise for a person with Alzheimer's. Eventually the benefit of exercise will become evident as fingers and hands get stronger. Help with starting the unwinding if necessary. Unwound twine can be used in other activities such as decorating a basket or wrapping around a vase or bottle. Twine comes in various sizes—larger is, of course, easier to unwind than the thin, tightly-wrapped size.

Modified Bingo

Modified Bingo uses familiar names, places and things instead of numbers. It is easy for a person in early stages to use a large variety of words.

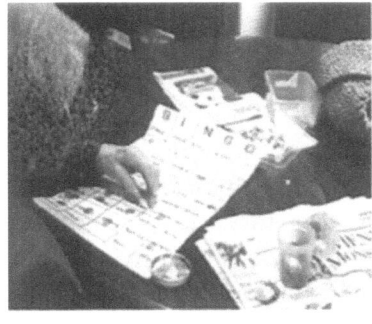

The names can be shorter in later stages. Choose the names and length of words that match the person's ability and interest. Each card can relate to a theme, eg. sports, hobby, work, etc. Use words associated with basic needs or likes such as foods, drinks, name of pet, names of family members, familiar street names, jewelry, tools, vacations, people, etc. In later stages, bingo cards can have fewer columns and fewer choices. Make bingo cards from letter-size craft paper with large squares so they are easy to see. As an example, under the letter "B" you can list ball, belt, boy, barber, banquet, bracelet, ballet, bush, bat, butter, bed, bread, blanket, butterfly or bubble. Long words may be too small to read if written or typed in the square. Continue this for each bingo letter. As you call out a bingo choice, you might say, "Look for 'bush' under 'B'." Rules for winning can be adjusted to accommodate the person's interest level or attention span. This game can be played with an individual or a group. To add interest, you can ask alert persons to spell the word once it is found on the card.

Word Games

Crossword puzzles, word search puzzles, and Scrabble

These are examples of word games that are designed for a wide variety of abilities. Most are available in large print format and are generally focused on a special area of interest, such as travel, game shows, movies, sports, or music. You can find games with themes related to information in the Personal Profile Form.

Word games are available that are designed for almost any level or ability. Carefully select games designed for a level appropriate for the skill level. When you find a word game the person enjoys, continue to use the same game or words until they recognize it as a game previously played. At that point, it is time to introduce a new game or increase the difficulty of the one they are playing. In later stages of Alzheimer's disease, you can ask the person to find a letter, rather than find a word.

Spelling

Spelling familiar words can be fun if letters are selected from a word game such as Scrabble. Choose names associated with positive experiences, such as hobbies, games, or from any other activity. The spelling game can be modified to match the person's skills. The most difficult skill level would require the person to select from a box of miscellaneous letters to spell a word. The words that you select can be adjusted for the skill level of the player. The game can be made significantly easier by limiting the letters you place in front of them to only the letters used in the word. All that would be required of the person is to arrange the letters to spell the word. If a player has difficulty spelling words, write the word on paper to make it easier for them.

Another variation to reduce complexity is to partially write the word on paper and supply only the letters to fill in the blanks. Begin at a level the person is comfortable with and continue to increase complexity as skills improve.

Identifying states and capitals

Most of us learned to identify states and capitals during our school years. Many with Alzheimer's might recall some or all of these names. Mentioning that you might be taking a trip to a particular state, but can't recall the name of the state capital, may stimulate conversation if the person is originally from that state. If the answer comes quickly and correctly, then follow through with conversation and see how the person responds. Another method to reduce complexity is to ask the question and offer a choice of two answers. Include choices that are easy to recognize as incorrect answers. Be sure to make it fun and casual. If it feels like a test, then the person could easily become discouraged.

Naming presidents

Because politics is such an important part of American life, talking about past or current presidents can stimulate political thoughts and conversations. Deeply embedded feelings can surface by asking about political preferences. Conversations about voting in elections can jog memories of politicians who were significant in the person's life.

Talking about politicians or political subjects may bring about fond memories or, on the other hand, may stir up very uneasy feelings. Don't take a political stance. Encourage the person to share thoughts without fear of being criticized or challenged.

Finishing famous sayings

Start a famous phrase, quote or proverb and have the person guess the missing word(s). For example:

What goes up _____ (must come down).
Don't put all of your eggs in _____ (one basket).
Early to bed, early to rise makes a man _____ (healthy, wealthy and wise).
If someone is having difficulty remembering the entire phrase, decrease the number of words you ask for. Instead, say "What goes up must come _____ (down)" or "A penny saved is a penny_____ (earned)."

If the person does well guessing the missing word, use phrases requiring more than one word to complete. On the other hand, if they struggle with multiple word answers, use phrases that require a one word answer. If none of the missing words can be recalled from the famous saying, you can read the entire phrase to them to stimulate. Often, hearing a familiar phrase will stimulate memories associated with the phrase. As an example, if you say "Don't put all of your eggs in one basket", it may remind them of an Easter egg hunt when they were young or seeing their children or grandchildren put eggs in a basket. If they once lived on a farm, it may remind them of gathering eggs from the chicken coup. Eventually, some phrases will be remembered or recognized. During upcoming sessions, don't be surprised if they join in as you read the phrases.

Fun Activities

Visiting with children

Visiting with young children can often be calming to a person with Alzheimer's. Children have a way of disarming even the most uncooperative person with their nonthreatening approach. Nurturing is a natural response when visiting children. Spontaneous feelings of parenting similar to when their children were younger have a calming effect. They enjoy hearing the children's voices and hear them tell about school and other activities. Children can make you laugh. In later stages, a doll can provide some of the needs and comfort that children do. They retain the need to be a role model for the children and feel compelled to be on their best behavior while visiting with them.

Listening, singing and dancing to favorite songs

Listening to uplifting music from the past usually stimulates memories of enjoyable activities. Often songs are enjoyable because they remind the person of a special relationship or memorable event. The type of music the person enjoys (show tunes, polkas, classical, religious) are listed in the Personal Profile Form. If you show interest in moving to the beat of the music, it often encourages the person to express their own feelings and be inspired to sing or dance. If the person stands up to dance, position yourself nearby to provide assistance if needed.

Plant seeds indoors or outdoors

Watching plants grow from seeds is a great experience for everyone, especially persons with Alzheimer's. They take great pride in seeing the sprouts grow due to their care. Supply seeds that have a high success rate. Check the plant during each visit to make sure it is being watered. You may want to water the plants, but certainly it is more rewarding if the person can handle this responsibility. If the person is feeling down and needs some cheering up, you can produce positive results in a short period of time by bringing in shoots or seedlings that have already sprouted.

Coloring or painting pictures

Many enjoy seeing results of their coloring efforts. They can use colored pencils or watercolors (depending on their abilities) to draw whatever they please, even scribbled lines, and select the colors for pictures they have drawn.

If the person does not like a certain color, remove that color beforehand and provide pictures that require colors they like. If you don't know their favorite colors, blues and pastels generally have a calming effect, and light ones rather than dark ones can lift one's spirit and mood.

Those who can't draw, can color pictures from paint by numbers or an adult-theme book of favorite subjects. Encourage them to stay within the lines as best as they can. If it is difficult for the person to hold a brush, crayon or pencil, they may enjoy using finger paints. The paint and aroma can stimulate thoughts of earlier experiences painting in school or at home with other children. For those who enjoy painting, this activity can be most relaxing. If your loved one doesn't want to paint for fear of making mistakes, start the painting and ask for his/her help. Painting together helps reduce the fear of making mistakes. You can help guide the brush if they are having difficulty. Allow the person to do as much as they are able to. You can help fill in the finer details yourself to complete the picture. Sharing a good time with you will make them feel special. After a few sessions they will gain enough confidence to complete a project without your help.

Playing cards

Most persons have played card games either as a child or an adult. A person with Alzheimer's may still be able to play a full game, or may only be able to recognize features of the cards, e.g., numbers, suits or colors. Card games can be modified to make them easier to play. Card games are usually fun for most persons at some level.

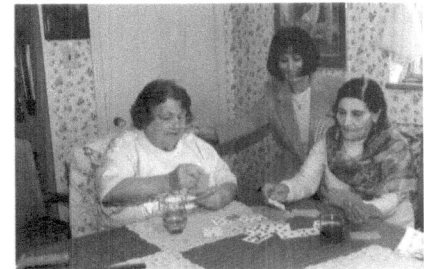

Make up your own simple games such as arranging by suits, colors, value, etc. Even shuffling or stacking the cards can be beneficial.

Working a simple puzzle

If puzzles are matched to the person's skill level, and have good color definition, they can be both a challenging and rewarding activity. Usually puzzles containing no more than 18-24 pieces are within most skill levels. Choose adult-theme pictures rather than cartoon or young children's puzzles.

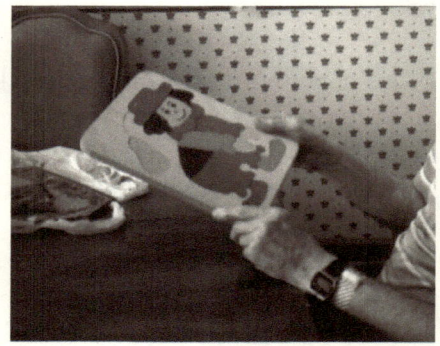

If they liked golf, a puzzle with a golf theme would be well received. If they enjoy being outdoors, try a nature-theme puzzle; if they like pets, an animal puzzle would be appropriate. Any theme associated with a past hobby, skill, or fun experience may be motivating.

Pet activities

Pets can be very entertaining for a person who has enjoyed caring for pets in the past. Not all care facilities will allow pets on their grounds, and any visits with animals must be approved by the staff. Animals must be friendly, calm and obedient. Usually, smaller dogs are better choices. A person can get an emotional boost and a feeling of being in control when a pet responds to a command. For persons who may not be comfortable with larger animals, fish, birds, guinea pigs or other pets that can be confined in a small space may be appropriate. They require very little care and are not very demanding of person's time. A bird can be entertaining, but certainly requires more work than fish. If the person is unable to take care of a pet at home or in the facility, arrange to bring pets in periodically. A visit to a pet store will allow the person to enjoy seeing pets, and give you a chance to observe what may be appropriate to use in activities that include a pet theme.

Cutting designs from greeting cards, magazines, or self-made designs

Greeting cards provide many different subjects for conversation with you. A Christmas tree ornament can be created by putting a string through a cut out picture. For Valentine's Day, hearts could be cut from cards and used to decorate the living area. Compiling a notebook or collage of different cutouts from cards of past holidays and special events might be fun. On St. Patrick's Day, one can color and/or write names on pre-cut shamrocks.

Tracing shapes on a plain piece of paper is a stimulating exercise, particularly if the shapes used are within the person's ability. Use simple geometric shapes you might find on familiar items such as coins, a drinking glass, bowl, other small items, leaves, star shapes, or cookie cutters. The person may want to decorate the picture with favorite colors before cutting it out. This activity is easily adjusted to the person's moods and abilities. Pictures can be taped to walls, hung as a mobile with a string, or displayed on a table.

Taking a ride

Many at any stage of Alzheimer's disease usually look forward to a trip in the car. As the disease progresses, they become more and more homebound with fewer opportunities to go outside. In time, they become more isolated and begin living like a "shut in." Even a ride around the block is a treat for some. Many enjoy the feeling of freedom that comes from getting away from their everyday environment. Prior to any trip away from the home or facility, always refer to the "Important Guidelines" at the beginning of this chapter for medication or medical conditions that may pose a health or safety risk. Remember to obtain permission from a facility director before leaving the facility's premises. A person with Alzheimer's who is away from their familiar environment might be afraid of getting lost. Keep your focus and attention on the person 100% of the time.

- Usually they appreciate visiting favorite places (parks, landmarks or restaurants). This could stimulate good memories. Often just seeing familiar sights again promotes recollection of people or events.

- Garage sales are often a source of enjoyment and may stimulate conversation about items they used to have or reasonably-priced pictures they may like.
- A trip to the ice cream shop is always a treat. Try to engage in conversation whenever appropriate.
- If a person with Alzheimer's used to love horses but cannot ride any more, improvise by going on a buggy ride, to the horse races, to a stable where horses are being groomed, rent movies about horses, or find news or magazine articles about famous horses.

Dyeing Easter eggs

A person with Alzheimer's may view dyeing eggs as a child's activity. If the eggs are being painted for use at a children's Easter egg hunt, it will help them feel useful and enjoy helping you prepare the eggs. Since painting eggs is typically a family affair, offer to invite a family member to join in the activity. Another option is to put the finished eggs into a decorative basket and donate it to a charitable organization.

Stringing Cheerios to hang outside for the birds

Usually a person will feel a sense of accomplishment after successfully creating something the birds enjoy eating. Cheerios have large holes, and are fairly easy to string. Threading the string through each cheerio and tying a knot between each one requires careful concentration and can improve hand/eye coordination. The string of Cheerios can be hung on a tree limb, fence, or wrapped around a stick and pushed into the ground.

Identifying pictures

Show pictures or cards and ask what is liked or disliked about them. Let them explain the meaning of the picture in as much detail as possible. If pictures are easily recognized, spelling some of the words related to the pictures may be appropriate. Provide clues if needed. The pictures will be more easily recognized if they are familiar scenes. It is not important to read the text, but rather to understand and react to the feelings generated by viewing them.

Recommended magazines include *National Geographic*, outdoor sports, entertainment, people-focus, or travel. When looking at nature pictures,

Amira C. Tame, A.C.C.

be sure there are no pictures that could upset the person with Alzheimer's. Pleasant pictures can have a calming effect.

Playing yard games

- Horseshoes is a stimulating activity and has simple rules that can be easily explained. Whoever lands the horseshoe closest to the pin is awarded the point. This game can be played with safe, rubber horseshoes and wooden pegs that could be installed anywhere in the yard. The game can be adjusted to make it more difficult or easier (put the pegs closer or farther apart). If rubber horseshoes are not available, use a ring toss game, that can easily be played indoors or outdoors.
- Another yard game is croquet, that is also easy to adjust to varying abilities. Once the person learns the rules, you can make the necessary adjustments, such as placement of wickets. The game can be as simple as placing one wicket in the grass and using the mallet as you would a putter in golf.
- Badminton or volleyball (using a soft ball) is also fun and provides a little exercise and, hopefully, stimulates conversation.

Indoor sport games

- If a pool table is available, pool can be a relaxing activity. It doesn't require prior knowledge of the game, and the rules are simple. It doesn't matter if the person is playing the game well. Just holding the stick and making contact with the ball can be very exciting and challenging. Pool can be played with a full rack of balls using regulation rules, or simply by striking a ball with the cue stick. There is no pressure to make the balls go into the pockets. Pushing the balls into the pockets by hand is also fun.
- Table tennis is another activity that can be played with rules adjusted to the skill and interest level. With the table against a wall you can bounce the ball against the wall and it will return.
- Putting a golf ball on a mat with a hole at one end and trying to get the ball inside the hole is a great game. If an automatic ball return is available, it will simply roll the ball back to the player and save some steps. It is stimulating for the player to watch the ball come right back out. The automatic ball return provides a bigger

target and the incentive for putting well is to see the ball return. Stand close to the person during the putting activity so you can support them if they become unsteady while putting the golf ball. A lightweight practice golf ball can be substituted for a real one to make this activity safer. This low impact activity may trigger thoughts of a round of golf or a shot that was especially memorable. Golf is a sport that is usually filled with exciting moments and provides an opportunity to socialize with friends.

- Indoor bowling can be played with lightweight plastic pins and a lightweight plastic ball. Set the pins a comfortable distance away. If you are concerned about the person falling, arrange the pins so one does not have to leave their seat to bowl. Show enthusiasm when any pins are knocked down. Practicing this activity usually results in improved performance. Even a slight amount of improvement can provide a great deal of satisfaction.

Making homemade ice cream treats

Creating ice cream desserts can bring back memories of when the person with Alzheimer's was young and ice cream was a special treat. The Personal Profile Form indicates the person's preference in ice cream flavors, and as with any food, whether or not ice cream is allowed in their diet.

You can work together to make an ice cream sundae by encouraging the person to peel and slice a banana, chop nuts, dice small pieces of fruit, and assemble the items in the dish. Another ice cream treat could be a milkshake made in a blender. If the person is allergic to milk, you can freeze favorite juices or soda pop flavors in Popsicle molds.

Making holiday cards

Holidays are a good time to share memories of family gatherings. Most holidays are memorable celebrations shared with loved ones and friends throughout one's lifetime. Many holidays or special days, such as birthdays and anniversaries, are expressed with cards containing verses that help the giver express positive feelings. For a person with Alzheimer's, feelings are easier to remember than factual details. Greeting cards provide a great opportunity to express feelings to loved ones. Keep a list of birthdays for which the person may want to make a card. It always makes them feel good to let others know they remember the occasion. If making a card from scratch is too difficult, a special message can be written on a store bought card. If there is no one to celebrate birthdays with, you can celebrate your own birthday with the person. Their birthday is certainly a special day to celebrate, especially if you bring a card with a special birthday message.

Preparing a holiday pumpkin

In this activity, a person with Alzheimer's helps prepare for Halloween. Use a plastic fruit and vegetables knife to cut the pumpkin and clean out the inside. The feel and aroma of the pumpkin can bring back memories of trick-or-treat days or Halloween festivities. A face can be drawn or painted on the pumpkin instead of cutting holes.

This is a very useful activity to help connect persons with grandchildren and stimulate conversations about childhood experiences.

Feeding animals

Feeding animals can be a rewarding experience because it makes one feel close to nature. Seeing the animals eat the food gives them a feeling of doing a good deed. They enjoy knowing the animals will come to them to be fed. Discourage feeding aggressive animals like swans and geese. Usually smaller animals such as squirrels, chipmunks, ducks and birds are safe to feed.

Arranging flowers

This activity brings back memories of happy times. Flowers typically are a reminder of Spring, warmer weather, and green grass. Refer to the Personal Profile Form to learn which flowers the person likes and is not allergic to. Fresh flowers help recall certain aromas and stimulate recollection of related events.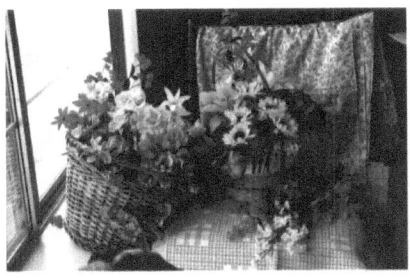

If you are unsure of allergies the person with Alzheimer's has, artificial flowers may be the better choice. Arranging flowers provides an opportunity to be creative and feel good about the project. The arrangement can be given to someone special who comes to visit, or it can remain in the room so the person can continue to enjoy and show it to others.

Tangle Yarn

Untangling yarn or twine is a task many people are familiar with. If you sense that the person you're working with is not interested in doing any activity, ask for help to unravel your tangled yarn. Usually a person is willing to help you with your problem, for a change. The tangles can be more complex for early stage Alzheimer's and as simple as winding yarn on a spool in later stage. Prepare the ball of yarn for this activity in advance. Many knots can be prepared that are easy to untangle, such as slipknots or bow-knots, etc. If untangling is too difficult of an activity, you can untangle the yarn while the other person winds it on a spool. This activity does not have to be finished in one session. It's easy to put away for another day.

Sorting familiar (sewing box) items

Most households have a sewing box full of odds and ends like bows, thread spools, buckles, bobbins, safety pins, snaps, buttons, paper clips, thimble, tape measure, etc. Men may prefer such items as keys, small hand tools, hardware items, golf balls, golf tees, nuts, bolts, washers. Items may be sorted by size, shape, or color. They may be able to describe the items and their uses, spell the names of the items, or describe instances when they have worn or used the items. Sorting and identifying the items provide opportunities for conversation. The simplest form of sorting would be to sort different colors of the same object into various containers, each container having only one color. Colored marbles or beads can be sorted in a certain order. You can place the first set of marbles in the order you choose (e.g., red, yellow, blue) in a straight line and ask the participant to repeat the pattern. They can also be beads on a string.

A more difficult activity is to mix plastic, wood or metal items of different sizes and sort them into associated groups, such as sewing items, jewelry, tools or golf items. Sorting by material (e.g., plastic, wood or metal) may be easier for some. These same familiar items could also be used for other games and activities that may stimulate memories of past activities.

Sorting coins

Often a person with Alzheimer's can recognize coins that have been used as money since childhood. Coins can be sorted by value and/or size.

If there are 50 of any particular coin, they can be counted and put in coin wrappers. If you bring a jar of coins, they may enjoy helping you sort them. During this activity, concerns about the person's personal finances may surface. Give reassurance that those finances are safe.

It is easy to see the progress made with this activity as the jar is emptied and the number of rolls increase. After rolling, the various rolls can be sorted and counted. Encourage participation at whatever level they can without becoming frustrated. If the person is able to count the money, let them keep track of their progress on paper for you. If there is a large amount of assorted coins, you can use an inexpensive coin counting machine to help with the task.

Making wood projects

This is an excellent activity in that the participant can produce products that can be used in other activities. Many pre-cut projects designed for a wide variety of skill levels are available at craft or hobby shops. Some examples are:

- An unfinished wooden bowl can be sanded until it is smooth.
- Assembling a predrilled magazine rack using wood glue is easy and can be used by the person when completed.
- Favorite pictures can be put into pre-cut picture frames that require assembling, gluing and clamping. It is safer to use plastic sheets cut to size to protect the picture instead of glass.
- A loom and hook board using small nails and a pre-marked board can be made to use in the loom activity, or can be used by others.
- Pegboard material can be cut to various shapes and used to place colored marbles on to create a pattern or picture.

Family Video

Make a narrated video of family members. Ask the family members to reminisce about the good relationship they had with the person. They should mention any memorable events. Seeing and hearing loved ones and friends talk about feelings and experiences from their past helps them remember the good old days and may stimulate more memories.

Treasure Hunt

Treasure Hunt consists of seeking, finding, and identifying buried treasure. Bury familiar items, such as rings, coins, dice, keys etc. in a bowl of colored sand or rice.

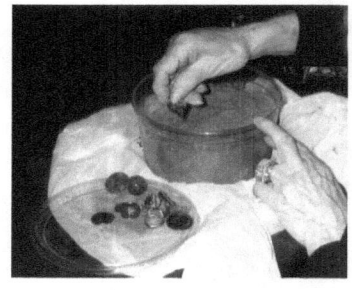

Using items they were familiar with in their past will help make this activity interesting. The object of this activity is to find an item in the bowl of treasures and identify it by feel, and then by looking at it. If the object is still not recognized, give hints such as where it's worn or what it sounds like.

Before looking for another treasure, you can say what it is. Let them know it's O.K. if they don't recognize all of them. Put each item that was difficult to identify back in the bowl, after you tell them what it is. They may be able to recognize certain items after finding them and hearing the names several times. For persons alert and able to recognize all, or most of the items, spelling their names can provide another stimulating challenge.

If the person doesn't like putting their hands in the bowl, you can still do the activity by looking for items yourself and identifying what you find. Touching, seeing and spelling the names of the items may trigger memories associated with them (e.g., a special broach or ring, a significant event or gift). This activity provides not only physical (hand and finger exercises) but also hand/eye coordination and memory recall stimulation. Treasure Hunt is fun and encourages participation in other activities.

Cloth/materials

Prepare three pieces of material (approximately one square foot) of different colors and textures. Number each piece 1, 2 or 3. There are many ways for the person to benefit from this activity. Patterned material may remind them of a favorite item or event. Distinctions between the pieces of cloth (texture, color and number) stimulate associative recall. Ask what color they like best, which piece of cloth feels the best to them or what color is the smoothest piece of cloth, etc. They may associate the color, texture or pattern with the number. Some associate materials with articles of clothing, table cloths, bed linens, upholstery, blankets, etc. Memories of shopping, decorating or special events may be triggered. The material can have distinct contrasts of textures and colors. Textures can vary from potato sack to fine silk and from plastic to knitted pieces. The more stark the contrast between colors and texture, the easier it is to distinguish the difference.

Pigeon hole box

This activity can be made from a box with compartments such as are used to separate glass items. The box can be placed on its side in which small items can be inserted to a comfortable depth. Openings should be numbered so the person can distinguish one compartment from another. Study the Personal Profile Form beforehand to determine types of items that may be recognized and use some of those items for this activity. The items placed in the openings may be familiar items used with other games. Ask the person to reach into the various openings until an item is found. Ask if the item looks familiar. The player may be able to spell the name of the item and/or remember which numbered compartment it was removed from. As ability improves, you can put items in more openings. Make this activity as challenging or simple as needed to benefit the person with Alzheimer's.

Make note of where the items are placed so you can put them in the same compartments. During the learning stages, put the same items in the same numbered hole to reduce complexity. Let the person put the items away to help them recall where to find them the next time you use this activity. You are more apt to recall the route in unfamiliar areas if you are the driver rather than the passenger.

Chinese checkers or marble art

This game can be easily broken down into different skill levels. A Chinese checker board consists of 6 triangles around the perimeter of the board and each triangle has small depressions where marbles can be placed. The colored marbles used match the colored sections. For one activity, sort the marbles by color and place them on the matching color on the board. This could progress to actually playing the game of Chinese checkers. A variation of this game could be utilizing a blank, square or round board (a piece of large-holed peg board may work well).

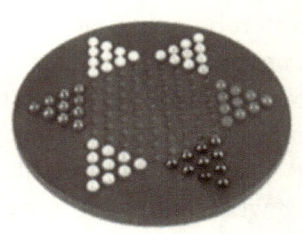

You could also use a dish strainer with perforated holes useful for a free form of Chinese checkers. Work as a team initially to demonstrate how the colored marbles can be used to make unique designs. Eventually, many will begin to feel comfortable creating their own designs on the board without fear of failure. Placing the colored marbles in a row with either the same color or in a repeating pattern can be used as a low function activity.

Familiar Sights and Sounds

Video tape sights and sounds that are recognizable. Pictures and taped sounds may be used to connect sight and sound as well. Play the sound and repeat it as many times as necessary to help stimulate memory through sound recognition. If the player cannot identify the sound, show the video and sound together. Give hints if necessary. The sounds you select should be ones they have likely heard in the past. Examples are:

- clock ticking
- dripping water
- material or paper being torn
- cup of coffee or dish being broken
- ocean waves
- washing dishes
- bathroom shower

- closing a window or door
- lawn mower
- electric saw
- cars or motorcycles driving by
- beeper
- vacuuming
- typewriter key sounds

Amira C. Tame, A.C.C.

Mixed Number Recall

This activity can help improve memory recall and build self confidence. The player looks for a number in a deck of colored cards that you prepared in advance. Each color corresponds to a level of difficulty. As an example, on the yellow you can put single digit numbers; on the blue cards, double digit numbers; on the red cards, three digit numbers, etc. The key is to make sure the number of digits, and location in the deck is an appropriate skill level. Make sure the cards are large unough to handle (approx. 3"x3") and the numbers are large and bold. The numbers can be put on with a wide felt marker. The object of the game is for the player to look for a number that is on one of the cards in the deck. The deck will have a mix of numbers and colors that is appropriate for the player.

In early stages, they may be able to find any number, located anywhere in the deck, and you can use all of the colors. In later stages, begin with single-digits placed within the first few cards, so they can be found on the second or third try. Success with the easy ones will encourage continued participation. Each time a number is located, place the next one further 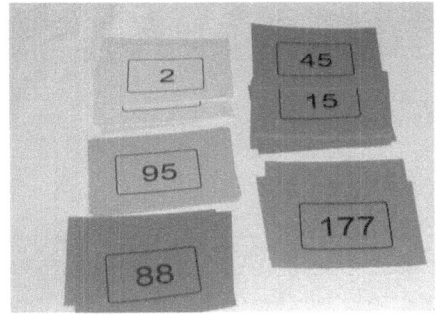 into the deck. Fit the activity to the player's ability by placing the card far enough into the deck to be challenging but not frustrating. The object of this activity is to look at the cards one at a time until the number you asked them to look for is found.

As the disease progresses, it may become more difficult to recall a specific number or color. A player may be able to progress to more difficult colors, as skill level and confidence improves.

This activity is one that can provide positive reinforcement and stimulate memory function at the same time.

The key to success in this activity is making sure the size of the number, e.g., one, two, three or more digits, and where you place the number in the deck is appropriate for the player's ability.

This activity, specifically designed to provide direct feedback of memory function, can be very beneficial if administered properly. On the other hand, negative results may ensue if it is too difficult. After several unsuccessful tries, remove the difficult card before the next session. It is important that a player be able to locate the numbers within the deck.

Regardless of the number of cards in the deck, ask for the same number each time, so it will be easier to remember for a longer period of time. When it becomes easy to find, it is time to place the card deeper into the deck or change the number to a more difficult one.

As the numbered card is moved deeper into the deck it requires remembering the number for a longer period of time. Again, stick with the same 2-digit numbers until you can increase to 3 digits. The goal is to remember the number as long as possible and progressively increase the number of digits remembered.

Family Connection

On 3x5 cards, write the names of family members or friends and their relationship to the person with Alzheimer's. If you have a photo, attach it to the back of the card. Seeing the photo associated with the name might help stimulate memories when that person visits and help to recall the visitor's name. You can determine, by referring to the Personal Profile Form, which relationships are appropriate for this activity. The relative's or friend's names that you use on the cards must be ones you know they like.

Find out as much as you can about each person from loved ones and family members before the session. Their input can help with the recall exercise. Family members may include special pets or special friends. You may include your name as a friend or caregiver, or whoever the person is most likely to view you as. Each card can have its own color. The color of the card associated with the name may help the player remember the relationship.

As an example, on one card you might write, "Claudia is my aunt." On another, you might write, "Amy is my friend."

Have the player read the cards one at a time. As each card is read some memories may stimulate conversation about that person, or relative to their relationship with that person. It is important to use names of relationships that won't trigger negative feelings. Talk about that one card and the person who was special. Taking turns reading the cards may help relieve tension. Tell them it's O.K. if they don't recognize the name or picture on the card. Let them know that this activity is designed to help them. As the relative's name becomes easier to recall, add another card so more relationships can be remembered. If the player is unable to recall anything at all about any cards, put the cards away for another time. Eventually, memories of relationships may be stimulated by other activities, and you can return to this one with more success.

Mood for the Day

Mood for the day can draw feelings and moods from an otherwise non-verbal activity session. Often, victims of dementia have lost confidence in their ability to communicate needs or feelings. Some are afraid to express real feelings, or feel that nobody really cares or understands. They may not want to risk hurting another person's feelings by saying what they think or feel. Many times, the ability to put feelings into words is locked away in lost memory. The sentences on the magnetic cards include many of the common feelings that are difficult to express for many elderly people. Don't say that this activity is intended to help express one's mood. Doing so, may create an emotional roadblock, and inhibit free expression.

Make 20-30 magnet moods with print that is large enough for them to read. (I use self adhesive blank magnetic business cards and a metal cookie tray that the magnets can stick to). Use only enough cards at one time that will provide a selection without being confusing. With some residents I use 10-12 cards, and with others I use only two at a time.

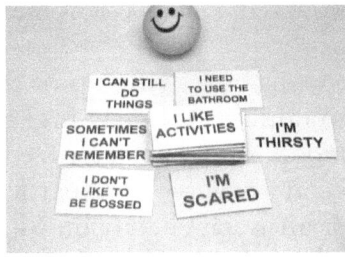

Print statements that express thoughts, feelings or emotions, e.g., I love you, I feel down, I want out of here, it's a beautiful day, I have a good family, I miss my dog. Each should be attached to the magnetic card. Some are happy feelings and some are not, but all of them are real and need to be expressed.

Place the cards randomly, face up on the inverted lid of the activities kit (or other tray) to make them easy to see and pick up.

Ask the player to pick out the ones that are their favorite. Allow time to ponder the choices without any pressure from you. Continue until several proverbs are selected. The player may be willing to express thoughts about the proverbs that can help you understand feelings that they had not been able to express.

Ask if they would like to keep one magnetic note on the refrigerator or another place. If the choice is to keep or display the mood card, it could mean that they want to share this feeling with a family member or another person. Leaving the tray of proverbs in their room may stimulate new thoughts for another session. At the next session, observe if one or more of the selected proverbs had been selected at a previous session. Proverbs that are repeatedly selected may have some significance.

The KEY element of this activity is feelings were expressed that may not have been without the help of this activity. Keep notes to see if a pattern emerges that might indicate a mood or issue that you may be able to help resolve or work around. Proverbs repeatedly selected may have some significance.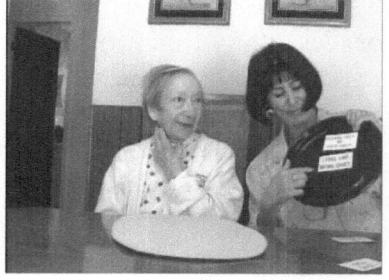

Moods can swing up or down from day-to-day or, sometimes, minute to minute. You may find a common factor that will lead to normalized mood swings or improved behavior. These trapped feelings may have been a roadblock to participation in activities or the source of resistant or antisocial behavior. Mood For the Day is a way to extract locked-in feelings without having to say the words and have fun too.

Wash a Car

Offer to help with washing his or her own car, a son or daughter's car, or any vehicle you have permission to wash. Begin the car washing process by gradually letting the person participate. This activity not only provides a feeling of being useful, but is an opportunity to get some fresh air on a beautiful day. Memories of when and where they drove or traveled in a car can be stimulated by this washing exercise.

Hide and Find

Use familiar items such as dice, coins or jewelry to hide under paper cups or bowls. Number each cup (possibly up to six different cups) and place an item under each one. You can progress from one item under one cup to more items under several cups. Be sure to use the same items each time you do this activity. In early stage, the player may want to spell the names of items as they find them.

Playing Music

This activity can be uplifting and often stimulates enjoyable memories and conversation. Songs from the past can bring back memories of a special relationship or a memorable occasion. They may want to sing or hum with the song. Music, such as show tunes, jazz, blues, classical & religious all have a long history, and may be beneficial.

Famous artists are often remembered in later years. Bing Crosby, Frank Sinatra, Kate Smith and Ella Fitzgerald are just a few. Family members and friends can help identify them. If you show interest by responding positively to the music with body language, it will encourage the person to express feelings. Just humming is sometimes helpful. Instruments can be used to stimulate interest by providing interaction with the music. Often, a person that was musically inclined may still have enough rhythm to keep time with the music.

You can use a tambourine, shakers, drums or any improvised instrument that can be used to make a sound. If they played piano as a child, they may still remember how to play a simple tune. You don't have to be a Tchaikovsky to have fun. I saw this proverb on a wall, in a restaurant. "A friend has a song in my heart, and sings it to me when my memory fails." Take time to enjoy music in your life too, and always keep a song in your heart. Music can also help you recall good times in your life, and help you through difficult times. Music can be a healer of wounds and relieve frustrations of the very difficult task of caregiving.

Scarf Toss to Music

Play familiar lively music or songs. Toss shear clothe in the air and catch it to the rhythm of the music. You can also toss the clothe in a circle to each other. Make the activity more exciting by using bright colored clothe.

This activity is fun, relaxing and help reduce anxiety. It also promote social interaction and may bring back happy memories of sewing projects.

Picture Card

Many individuals have played card games as a child or an adult. Person with early stage may be able to play a full game of cards or at later stages may only be able to recognize pictures on a card. Some games have funny cartoon animals and their names on the cards. Or you can create your own cards using familiar pictures printed on paper. There is 4 cards of each picture in a deck.

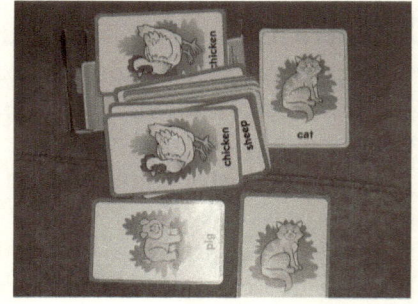

You can remove one of the cards and ask them to find a matching card in the deck. Because there are three identical cards left in the deck, they will have several opportunities to find the matching card. In the early stage you can show them the card and place it face down on the table. You can use many sets of cards for them to choose from. In later stage, you can hold the card so they can see it while they are looking for the matching card. You will use fewer card sets depending on their ability.

Low cognitive function individuals who may not be able to recognize words or identify numbers may be able to match pictures. Being able to match picture cards may give them self confidence to participate in other activities.

Home Tools

Home tools work especially well for anyone who made repairs around the home or who worked in a repair field. An activity using plastic plumbing and miscellaneous tools, such as, a tape measure, paint brush, lumber crayons, or square may stimulate memories of home projects. Some may be proud of accomplishments and are willing to talk about them.

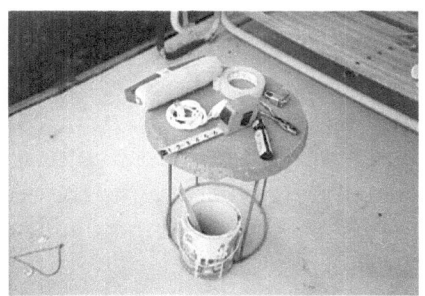

Plastic plumbing can be purchased in a variety of sizes and shapes. Many interesting projects can be constructed by connecting ones that fit. This activity can strengthen fingers and hands, improve wrist movement and stimulate memory recall.

Colored plastic nuts and bolts come in a variety of thread sizes and types. Removing the nuts from bolts that you have threaded will be easier for low function individuals. These activities will help strengthen fingers and hands, improve wrist movement, coordination and focus.

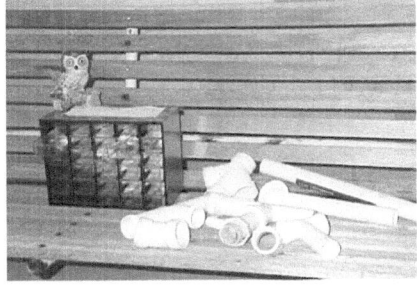

Number Recognition

Use a calculator that has a large type display. Show the player a handwritten number on a card or sheet of paper. Demonstrate how that number can be entered on the calculator. They may want to try to enter a number after watching you. Begin with single digits and gradually proceed to larger numbers. Improved number recall will be easily to recognize during this activity. A person in early stage dementia may be able to use the calculator to add, subtract or multiply to help with simple arithmetic problems.

Tying Ribbons

Ribbons can be tied in a variety of ways. You can tie simple half knots, full knots, single or double bows. The complexity of tying can be modified to their ability. The most effective approach is to begin tying the bow on his/her fingers. The person will pay closer attention if involved in the tying, rather than just watching you. It's always easier to learn if you are part of the process. Wrap the ribbon gently around extended fingers and lightly tie a single knot. Eventually, he/she may want to try tying a bow on your fingers.

Using favorite colors and material will help stimulate interest and help build self-confidence. Eventually, the participant may want to try to do it independently. Untying can be a part of the activity, and is also good for fingers and hands.

Loom Weaving

An inexpensive loom and hook kit can be purchased at a craft or department store or made out of a piece of wood as a separate craft project. A purchased kit has easy-to-follow instructions included.

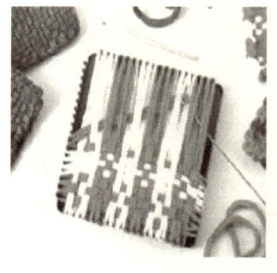

A loom can be made from a small piece of wood 8" square and 1/2- to 3/4-inch thick with small nails or screws evenly spaced around the outside edge. Extra bags of loops can be purchased separately. Items such as pot holders, coasters or a small mat can be created with favorite materials and colors. They are easy to make and can be useful as gift items. The elastic loops are placed over a pin and stretched to a pin on the opposite side. When all of the loops are attached in one direction, rotate the board 90 degrees and do the same thing by going over and under the loops you have already attached. If weaving is too difficult, the colored loops can be placed over each other in any fashion and still be admired as a piece of art. This activity also benefits fingers and hands, improves wrist movement, coordination, focus and may stimulate memories of times in their lives when they made woven projects.

Amira C. Tame, A.C.C.

Finding Numbered Items

Finding items in a box may become difficult as memory diminishes. Forgetting the names of once familiar items can be very frustrating and discouraging. Sometimes it's easier for them to remember short numbers long enough to find a numbered item. This activity can be used for any level of Alzheimer's and is beneficial, especially for individuals with low cognitive function.

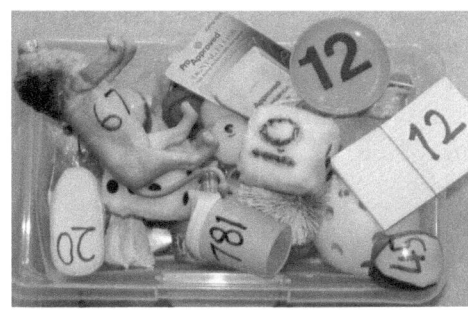

Print large numbers on familiar items or on a tag attached to them. Items should be large enough to be easily seen and light enough to be easily picked up. Names can be used instead of numbers on the items. This will not only help players find the item, but associating the printed name with the item will help memory recall.

You can include pictures of familiar faces with the names printed on the picture. Forgetting the names of loved ones can be delayed by including their pictures in this activity and using it often. This activity helps improve memory function without it seeming like a memory exercise. If you are not sure what to put on the tag, you can include both numbers and names. You can then use the method that works best for each individual.

Place the box of items within reach of the player, or at a distance that requires getting up from their chair and walking to the box if they can walk. Walking across the room provides exercise and increases the time required to remember the item. In a group, the box of items can be placed closer to persons with lower physical or cognitive function.

In earlier stages this activity can be challenging by dividing the players into small groups at separate tables. Each table will have a box of items in the center. Each member of the group is given one or more cards with the name and number of one or more items. Each card will correspond to an item in the box. At your signal, everyone looks for the item on their card. The table that finishes first can win a treat or a small prize. For a more orderly game, each table can begin with one person looking for an item before the next one looks. Continue around the table until all of the items have been found. If someone is having difficulty reading the card, the person sitting next to them may help.

Magnetic Wand and Chips

This is the newest of my activities. It is becoming popular because it's fun and challenging. The colored plastic chips have a steel ring around them that's attracted by the magnetic wand. The bright colors make this uplifting activity easy to modify to anyone's ability by varying the number of chips and variety of colors. I have a variety of ways to use this activity, and I'm sure that you can come up with many more too. My favorite one is to scatter chips on the table, and use the wand to pick up favorite colors without attracting others. It's possible for anyone, after a few laughs and many tries. Next, choose another color and try to pick them up without attracting the others. How many chips of the same color can you capture? Seeing that you are not able to collect very many chips will reduce the fear of failure. In later stages, just sorting and stacking colors may be enough to keep their interest.

Concentration, hand/eye coordination, motor skills, and reaction time can all improve with this activity. Remember, small articles can be a choking hazard!

Paper Twist

This activity uses tightly wrapped paper twine that was wrapped by a machine. Wrapping it was the easy part. The more difficult and most useful part of this activity is unraveling it. Start the unwinding process by straightening out one or two inches of twine and let them finish the job. This encourages participation.

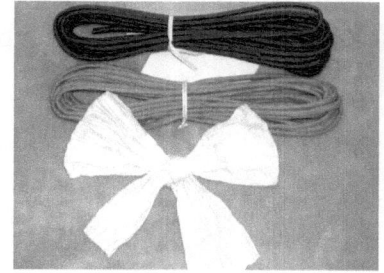

Selecting colors that interest the person in this activity is a key to willing participation. There may be colors you don't want to use because you know through other activities they are disliked by the participant. Cut the pieces of paper twist in short lengths (12-18 inches) so the task doesn't seem too large to accomplish in one sitting. Next, ask the participant to help you unwrap the paper twine into flat strips or ribbons of material so you can decorate a basket for a gift to a friend or a family member. If you work on one end of the piece while they work on the other they can observe how it's done. This gives a genuine feeling of doing something together, and, for a useful purpose.

This activity is popular, especially when the paper twine is to be used to wrap the handle of a basket of flowers just arranged. A bonus from participating in this activity is the hand and finger exercise that the person benefits from without calling it an exercise. It is especially useful for persons who are not interested in an exercise program, but are willing to help you with this project.

Chain Link

Colorful link chain comes with enough links to make a necklace and bracelet. The open links are easy to assemble and take apart.

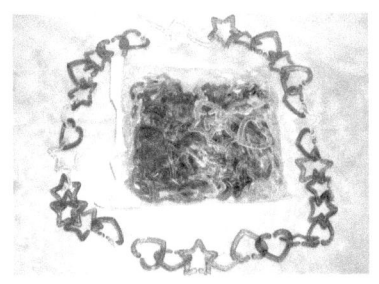

Hearts and stars shapes add a touch of love to the links. Always supervise activities that use small items which could be a choking hazard.

Magnetic Beads

Stringing beads can become difficult as eyesight and co-ordination diminish and can lead to added frustration for a person with Alzheimer's disease. With this activity you won't have to worry about the holes in the beads being too small to find. This activity does not require a string or holes in the beads.

There are no holes, and the string is a magnetic force that threads itself. You just move the marbles around, and they connect, just like magic. You can easily create many shapes. Another, more-demanding part of the activity is color recall. It can help identify favorite colors. Put any number of colored marbles on the table. Two or three may be all you can use in later stage Alzheimer's. In early stages, you can use a greater number of marbles and variety of colors. Ask the participant to select a favorite color. Remove the marble from the group and ask whether or not the one removed was the favorite one. If the activity is too easy, you can increase the number or variety of colors to make the activity more challenging. Another way to create a challenge is to ask the person to look at the colors very carefully, and then look away. While s/he looks away, remove a marble. Show the one you removed and ask if it was a favorite color. A correct answer is not as important as participation. Don't mention whether the answer was right or wrong. Just say, "Very good."

Again, you can determine the number of marbles and variety of colors, by observing ability and interest level. In later stage, color sorting and arranging simple designs may be challenging enough to make it fun and beneficial.

Favorite Jewelry

Sorting through a jewelry box and finding one to wear is fun and can bring back good memories and stimulate productive conversation. You can use costume jewelry that is easy to find in flea markets or second hand stores.

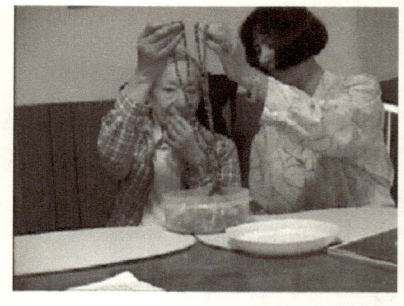

Using their own costume jewelry may trigger more memories of places they were worn or where they got them. Having a variety of colors will help you find out what their favorite colors are, and which ones they don't like at all. When they find one they like, tell them how pretty their choice is, and how beautiful they look when they try them on. With all of the negative things associated with their disease, it's not often they can get a compliment. Dressing up in something special and wearing special jewelry before going to a social can raise their spirits and improve their mood. They want to know that they can still look good when they dress up. Jewelry always seems to perk up attention and encourage participation in other activities.

NOTE: Always supervise activities that use small articles that can become a choking hazard.

Therapeutic Humor Activities

Balloon/Ring/Rubber Animal Toss

Tossing a rubber ducky and a rubber chicken around in a circle (instead of a ball) gets great laughs and provides exercise too. Balloon toss always gets everyone laughing. Use non-latex balloons if anyone is allergic to latex. Close-range ring toss gets players to participate because you can adjust the distance they must reach to match each of their abilities.

Folded Cards Charades

Another activity that gets a whole group laughing is to pass out folded cards with names of animals inside. I sit in the center of the circle and act out the animal sound after each reads theirs to me. In a low function group, they hand their card to me instead of reading it and when I make the sound of the animal I ask if anyone can tell me what animal it is. They don't have to worry about not recognizing it because I blame it in my poor imitation of the animal.

Egg Charades

Write the names of familiar sounds or things to do (sing, dance, jump rope, act out a sounds (train whistle, motor cycle sound, barking dog, etc.) on a card. Place a folded card into each plastic egg. Give each participant an egg.

Once all the eggs are distributed, ask everyone to open their egg and find out what action to act out. If a person can not act out his action they can trade with someone else. One at a time, each person will act out what is on the card and the rest of the group will try to guess what the note asked you to do.

Hand Puppet

Funny looking hand puppets are great because you can freely talk through the puppet without intimidating the person you're caring for and get great smiles. This technique is especially useful with individuals who are non-social or non-verbal. I've had clients who seldom show any emotion just break out laughing when they see my talking puppet. I have a variety of stuffed animals to help give them a reason to smile. Animated toys that talk can be fun or a way for them to express negative feelings if they don't like what is said without fear of hurting your feelings. After all, it was the toy that said it, not you. You can agree with their feelings to give them support.

Funny Classic Movies

Classic comedy movies are a great source of humorous situations that one can laugh at without following a complicated plot or story. Even silent movies can generate smiles. They were produced to be understood without the use of vocal dialogue. Subscripts and creative body language are very descriptive and leave room for individual interpretation. Sometimes reading the words on the screen is easier for some to understand than hearing the words. Some cartoons in newspapers are very humorous, even without words. Use political cartoons only if you know their political preference.

As with any activity, keep a record of what stimulates the person to laugh or smile, and the kinds of humor that doesn't. A personal profile record with this information can help you make humor a successful component in your activities program.

There is no greater gift you can give a suffering person than relief and hope. Your relationship with your loved one will improve as you stimulate positive memories and see his/her self-confidence, physical and mental abilities improve.

"When we bring sunshine into the life of others
We are warmed by it ourselves"

Amira C. Tame, A.C.C.

No one cares how much you know,
Until they know how much you care.

Hopefully, this book provides you with a systematic approach to reduce the emotional, functional and environmental effects of Alzheimer's disease through the use of these therapeutic activities and creative techniques.

The strongest emotional healers of wounds created by Alzheimer's disease are love, care and respect.

Alzheimer's was not brought on by anything you or your loved ones did or didn't do. So, be gentle with the person you are caring for and especially easy on yourself as you embark on this difficult journey. The emotional lift you will feel as you see your loved one benefit from this program will also help heal the wounds you may be suffering.

Chapter 7

Documented Case Histories of Clients' Improvements

I would like to dedicate this chapter to the many wonderful people I've had the opportunity of helping through a difficult time in their lives. I owe much of what I know to the experiences I've gained from seeing improvements in the people that I've had the opportunity to work with.

I've learned that with hard work and perseverance, you can improve the quality of life for the person you're caring for. These techniques and unique activities will make your work easier and more fruitful.

One's sense of humor is often the last sense affected by Alzheimer's disease and provides a momentary respite from the seriousness of other losses.

God bless you for caring and wanting to help.

Amira C. Tame, A.C.C.

In this chapter I share some personal experiences and interactions I've had with persons I've treated who were in various stages of Alzheimer's disease. You may recognize some of the methods and techniques described in previous chapters. Hopefully, you will find these examples useful to help you design your activity program.

Sophie's Story

When I began working with Sophie she was in the early stage of Alzheimer's, and living in a facility. Her face was filled with questions and confusion. She wasn't sure where she was, or why she was there. She insisted that she was still living at her home in Livonia and would be returning home soon. Her sister, who was in later stage Alzheimer's, was a frequent companion who shared activities I brought for Sophie. Stella could enjoy the same activity as Sophie at the same time, but at a different level. This shared interest kept Stella and Sophie close companions throughout their remaining years together. Often Sophie would question Stella about how she got to her home because she knew that Stella didn't drive any more. Of course Stella didn't have an answer. She would only answer in a frustrated voice, "How would I know; you must have brought me here." Neither realized that Stella lived in the room across the hall from her.

I couldn't let her know that I was an activities therapist, hired by their family to help her cope with her declining condition. I was simply a friend of her daughters who enjoyed spending time with her. This didn't cause any alarm or suspicion. My coming to see her was not only OK with Sophie, it made her feel good about me, and she even said "It's so nice for you to do this, God bless your heart." She felt very special when I came to visit her. I was not a threat, I was her friend. I was a source of news and a sounding board for her concerns about her family. Although her family visited often, she couldn't recall previous visits. The most repeated question I had to respond to was "When will my daughter be here," or "When is my son coming." Always the answer was, "They will be here soon." Sometimes Sophie would challenge me and ask "How do you know she's coming?" I would answer in the same way, "Because I just saw her today, and she said she would come today." This answer satisfied her question for the moment. I knew she would ask the same question many times before I was finished with the therapy session, and I would give her the same answer.

It's interesting to note that although Sophie could not remember visits by friends or family members, she never forgot the love she had for her family or the love they had for her. She often commented about how good her family was to her, and how good they were as persons. One of my favorite quotes is "They may forget what you say, they may forget what you do, but, they will never forget how you made them feel." Sophie needed answers. Where is she? Why was she here? How are her finances? How could she think about activities with all of these unanswered questions distracting her attention? Focused attention is difficult enough to muster without the clutter of unsettled confusion and unanswered questions. I knew where to begin with Sophie. I needed to build trust first, and then work on relieving her anxiety and frustration before it developed into fear and isolation. Sophie learned to trust me. After a few weeks of seeing Sophie, I explained that the home she had moved from was no longer safe for her. It needed a lot of work to make it safe, and it would cost a lot of money to do this. Her family was concerned about this, and decided that this was the best option. Eventually I drove Sophie to her old neighborhood and showed her the house she moved from. The house was still there. Somehow I sensed that from that day forward Sophie understood that she was in a better place.

It's time to try some activities other than conversation stimulation. I already know what Sophie likes to do. After all, our conversations weren't successful by accident. When I filled out her Personal Profile Form I found that Sophie's favorite subject in school was spelling. With Alzheimer's, long term memories are often retained through many stages of the disease. I was surprised that she wasn't afraid of misspelling words that I asked her to spell. They weren't all spelled correctly, but it didn't matter. She said that she felt proud that she could still spell difficult words. She wasn't aware that I was choosing words that I already knew she was familiar with. Again I referred to her Personal Profile Form that gave me clues as to the food, hobbies, entertainment, etc. that might trigger memories and spark an interest to participate in activities. Choosing activities and listening to music that she could relate to continued to enhance our developing relationship. When she would hear me play music from her past, it immediately got an excited response, "You've got to be kidding me. You mean that you like the same music that I do?" This just added fuel to our growing relationship. Sophie began to trust me more each session, and showed it by opening

Amira C. Tame, A.C.C.

up about her past and sharing feelings that were buried beneath a cloak of doubt and fear.

Sophie was not always in a good mood. She had mood swings like everyone else does. With Alzheimer's, the mood swings can be more dramatic and frequent than usual. They can swing up and down from day to day, and sometimes minute to minute. Sometimes Sophie just needed space. She never told me when she needed space. I needed to recognize the indicators that this was going to be a different session than the last one. It's important to be aware of the signs before the session changes to a negative experience. Flowers always brought a serene atmosphere to our activities session. Creating a beautiful bouquet from loose imitation flowers and greens always seemed to satisfy her needs while she was in a down mood swing. I kept notes in her progress report as to what usually worked as rescue activities when nothing else seemed to. It's important to adjust your expectations for a session to the needs, mood and abilities that day. I found that suggesting a ride in the car sometimes was all she needed to perk up her interest. Again, I knew what stores she frequented before coming to the facility, where she once lived, how to get to her favorite park etc. She remembered all of the stores that we visited. Her favorite store was the pet store. I observed her reaction to the various pets she encountered. I didn't take long to confirm the information collected in her profile information. She cruised right past all of the cats, dogs, hamsters, fish tank, and directly to the beautiful singing birds. This information helped stimulate many conversations and produce big smiles.

Sophie also wanted to stop in a textile store. She enjoyed showing me material and explained how she used to make clothes for her children when they were young, and proceeded to suggest what she thought would look good on me. As we drove through her old neighborhood, she pointed out all of the places she recognized. She was very excited and proud when she recognized the house she had lived in for many years. Stories were flowing as we passed a local park where she used to take her children. Sophie was tired now and ready to go home. She was in a much better mood. There was no right or wrong answers for Sophie's feelings or expressions. There was no threat of being wrong about anything. After all, who knows more about the places we visited than Sophie? A simple ride in the car turned a potentially unproductive activities session into a mind stimulating day for both of us. Sophie began looking at me as a real friend who cared about her and enjoyed her company. She felt that we shared so many interests. I think that she participated in some activities just because she liked me and felt that it would make me feel good.

Sophie liked jewelry very much, so I usually brought a container filled with old costume jewelry to our activities sessions. She liked sorting through the box and finding the ones she liked most. This also gave me an idea what her favorite colors are. I also occasionally took her to a garage sale on a nice summer day to look for inexpensive things to buy. I recall that I bought an old necklace at one of the garage sales. I didn't add it to my collection of jewelry for about six months. What convinced me that I was really making a difference for persons with dementia was when Sophie spotted the necklace in the box and said "This one looks familiar." I was shocked. After all, when I met Sophie, she had very little short term memory left. I said "Do you recognize it?" She said "Yes I do." I said, "We bought this at a garage sale this past summer. She paused for a few moments, as if in deep concentration, and "Yes I remember now." I was so excited I asked, "You do?" She said, "Yes I do, my brain still works. It's getting better now." I asked why she thought her brain was getting better and she said "Maybe it's because I have you now, and you see me a lot. Maybe it's because you care." "Maybe it's because we do things together." I asked what she liked to do. Her response was, "Anything." After a pause she said, "There's nothing worse than having nothing to do. It's awful being alone."

Lucille

Lucille was blessed with a husband who showered her with loving attention. But Lucille continually complained that her family was not "nice" to her. Neither her husband nor her children could do anything to please her.

When I first visited Lucille, she bluntly asked me what my "purpose" was in coming to see her. I told her that I was the friend she had been looking for. "You are?" she said. "You have to watch my husband and his family. They are greedy. They want my husband's money."

I told Lucille that her husband's family was also her family, that his daughters and sons were also her daughters and sons.

"No," Lucille said, "they are his kids, not mine, because they don't love me. They love only their father because he gives them money. They take advantage of him and they always take him out and leave me here."

John, speaking gently, said, "No, Honey, you always go with us when our daughters come over."

Seething with anger, Lucille glared at her husband and said, "I don't remember you ever taking me out. You are never with me. John, you have changed a lot lately. You don't care about me anymore." Then, reaching for her hand, he said, "Honey, I love you."

Enraged, Lucille exploded, "Get away from me!" Smiling sadly at his wife, John said nothing. John was suffering. He had cancer.

Time passed, but Lucille's anger remained. No matter what I did for her, she was not content. She wanted to be left alone and cried most of the time. I tried to figure out what was troubling her. So, After a week I thought to tell Lucille the story of a life filled with love and trust. Taking her hand gently in mine and looking steadily into her eyes, I told her of the great love and trust I feel for my husband and for his family.

Lucille listened quietly. When I finished my happy family story, she started to cry again. It was obvious that Lucille was not about to volunteer anything, so I asked her, "Would you like tell me what's bothering you?"

Angrily, she snapped, "Nothing. I don't know. I would like to go to bed and take a little nap."

Still seething with anger, Lucille went to bed. It seemed to me that she was confused, not tired. Perhaps by going to bed, she could avoid having to deal with what was troubling her.

She sat on her bed and I again asked, "Lucille, what is really bothering you?" Looking at me, she spoke quietly, "I can't even ask the question."

"Please ask," I said. "I think I may have the answer to your question and you might feel better." Lucille knew her husband would die soon, but this was not what was bothering her. Her great concern was, "Where is he going to be buried and will his family take me to his funeral?"

Crying, she told me, "His family (which is her family, too) will not let me know when John dies. What will happen to me after John dies? Is he going to leave me some money?"

I told her that, although I could answer her questions, her husband would be able to give her the best answers. She said, "How can I ask him these questions?"

I convinced her it would be okay to ask and that she should just sit next to her husband, hold his hand, tell him how she feels and ask him all the questions she has. I also assured her that I would be sitting next to her and she had nothing to fear.

Seemingly energized, yet calm, Lucille left her bed and seated herself next to her husband who was watching TV in the living room. Taking his hand, Lucille asked, "When you die, where are they going to bury you?" She started to cry.

Tenderly, John said, "Honey, don't worry. My grave is next to yours." She asked, "It is?" "Yes," he said. Then Lucille told him, "I want to die before you so I won't have to wait."

John tried to assure his wife further and said, "You will go to my funeral. When something is about to happen, you will know. Okay, Honey?"
I asked Lucille whether she had another question for John, and she said she did. Turning to John, she asked, "Who will be taking care of me after you die and how much money will you leave for me?" "Plenty of money," he told her.

Not satisfied, Lucille demanded that John tell her the exact amount. I told John she needs to know the amount of money, and after he told her the amount, her eyes opened wide. She relaxed and stopped crying.

I asked Lucille whether she had any more questions to ask John. She did not. Then, with her permission, I walked with her in the hallway and asked if she felt better. "Oh, yes I do," she said. She seemed to be relaxed and peaceful. Her attitude toward her husband changed from anger to peace and love.

John's health worsened, and he was confined to a wheelchair. One day, the nurse took him to his bedroom. He lay, mouth and eyes open. Lucille asked, "Oh, what has happened to John?" She said, "John, are you okay?" Looking at her, John answered, "No." Lucille knew that John was dying.

I told Lucille to hold John's hand and tell him that she loved him. Crying, she said, "He knows I love him." I said, "I know, but you had been angry at him lately. This is the time you need to tell him that you love him."

Guiding Lucille close to John's bed, I asked her to hold his hand and tell him everything she wished to tell. She held his hand and said," I want you to know that I love you." It was hard for John to talk, but he pressed her hand and said, "I love you, too."

Lucille stayed with John, holding his hands. She knew that John would be leaving her in a short while, and she cried. She felt better after expressing her love and care to him.

At John's funeral I asked Lucille how she was doing. She said, "I'm okay, but how can I make it without John?" Then she asked me to take her to the bank before anyone could take her money. I told her I couldn't take her until tomorrow. She complained that she didn't have enough money in her hand, so, to make her feel more secure, I gave her 10 one-dollar bills.

We went to lunch together and Lucille said she wanted to pay for lunch. She paid the cashier and received her change. She was happy. She was taking care of herself. She said, "I would like to move to a cheaper place, if I could, because I need to watch my money and be careful."

Helen

When I met Helen, she could not raise her arm or see well. She remained on a chair in the hallway and did not move. Saying nothing, I tuned to some classical music on the radio and sat next to her on the floor. I opened my brief case and started stringing some colorful beads, showing my progress from time to time. After about 20 minutes, she asked me what

I was doing. I told her I was trying to make a bracelet. She said, "I can see that. How do you do it?" I showed her how I was stringing the beads, and she said, "It's pretty. Can I have some beads to make a bracelet?" I said, "Sure. Let's do it together." We took turns putting beads on the string. After a while, she said she did not need help and finished the bracelet by herself. This activity was an icebreaker. After that, Helen changed from a disdainful client to a friendly person eager to chat with me about what was happening (or had happened) in her life.

On another day, however, Helen was obviously in a sour mood. I played classical music she had previously seemed to like. We listened together in silence for 15 minutes. Then I asked if I could sing for her. She said, "Yes," and I sang, but she did not join in. She looked quietly at some magazines I had given her. After a while, I asked her if she would pick up a yellow marble and put it on the tray. She picked up a green marble and said, "This is yellow." I said, "Okay. Put it on the tray." She then picked up an orange marble and said, "This is yellow." Finally, she selected a yellow marble and said, "This is yellow." I said, "The other marbles are green and orange. Why did you tell me they are yellow?" Helen said, "Because I like yellow, and I see them as yellow."

I wanted to cheer Helen because she still seemed to be in a bad mood. I had yellow, blue and pink clumps of play dough. I asked her to select one clump. She picked up the yellow play dough. I then asked her to squeeze the play dough in her hand and "take your frustration out on it." She started to squeeze the play dough, and she squeezed and squeezed, saying, "Eh, eh, eh . . ." Finally, she said, "Now I feel better. This is good exercise for my fingers." Helen is one of several clients who enjoy hand-finger exercises using play dough.

I realized that Helen retains a strong desire to control her life and those who affect her life. For example, I used to bring my brief case with me on visits to her. She objected to that brief case. Perhaps she thought it contained too many projects that she may not have wanted to work on.

Since one of my objectives is to help my clients retain a sense of independence and control over their lives, I now leave my brief case at home and carry in my purse what I need for a particular session. The next day when I came without my brief case I said, "See, Helen, today I do not have my brief case." She laughed with a triumphant expression.

Helen surprised me one day when she said, "Amy, my hands are feeling better. My right arm especially is much better. Thanks to you I can lift it up and move my fingers." Prior to my treating Helen, she thought she had lost the use of her right arm. In fact, she quit using her right arm for anything. I included simple flexing exercises in her activity program using her hands, arms, and fingers. Since Helen was convinced of her disability, she was not willing to participate in any organized exercises.

Allan

Allan's wife knows her husband's idiosyncrasies, one of which is asserting his independence from her when I am around. So, Allan's wife asked me to get him to take his medication. It was easy for me to get him to take his medicine because Allan likes the attention he gets from me. He is sure of his wife. After all, she has stayed with him for over half a century. Allan enjoys our times together and happily sings songs with me, arranges baskets of flowers, and does simple flexing exercises.

Allan's wife says that his excuse for not taking his medicine is he believes she is going to poison him. I think Allan just wanted extra attention from me. When I told Allan I could not give him his medicine because it was not part of my job, he took his medication from his wife without protest.

Allan tried to paint a picture, but he could not hold the paint brush. Instead, he decided that he would work with beads—blue, orange and white beads. He said his favorite beads were the white ones. When I asked him why he liked the white beads better than the others, he took off his shoes and put the white beads in his shoes. Then he put his hands in the shoes and said, "I feel good." He did this over and over again. Allan likes to participate in activities that he is physically capable of doing.

Ellen

My first session with Ellen began with her opening her front door and telling me I was not needed. Ellen is a very dignified and elegantly dressed woman who treasures her privacy and independence and resents any inference that she may be inadequate in any way. I resorted to coaxing—telling her I had made quite a trip to see her and asking her if she would let me in for a little while. Her innate sense of hospitality took over, and she admitted me into her home. That first session consisted mainly in Ellen sizing me up and both of us getting to know one another. The second session was quite different. She greeted me at the door, invited me in, walked to her chair, sat down, turned on the TV, and ignored me.

Ellen's son had talked to her and told her that he wanted her to participate in activities with the activity therapist. Ellen wanted to please her son, but she was not about to be told what to do by an activity therapist. Her son explained all this to me. So, respecting Ellen's feelings and giving her time to relax, I sat quietly for a few minutes. Then I started to comment on the TV program she was watching. She responded briefly, then continued to ignore me. I think she wanted me to leave, but she was too polite to say so. Subsequently, Ellen started to open up. She talked about each member of her family and expressed her love for them.

Ellen takes pride in her appearance and in her home. She makes certain that her outfits are coordinated and her hairdo is perfect. In line with her interest in clothes, I have presented her with material that she can cut and make into various sizes and shapes. She enjoys this quite a lot, and while she works, she talks. Ellen has proved to be a much more sociable person than her son had led me to believe. Not only does she tell me about herself and her family, she asks me about myself and my life—very much like any new acquaintance might. But, inevitably, a time comes during our conversation when she wants to say something and finds that she cannot remember a crucial word.

Forgetting where we have left something is an experience most people have. But when people afflicted with Alzheimer's disease forget where they have put something, we attribute their forgetfulness to their disease. Consequently, they may panic and frantically search for their misplaced possessions to avoid facing the possibility that they may be experiencing another symptom of this feared disease.

Amira C. Tame, A.C.C.

Fear of memory loss

One day Ellen couldn't find her purse. She became agitated and said, "Oh, my God. Where is my purse?" The more she searched, the more frantic she became. Nothing I said calmed her. Finally, I found her purse under her kitchen sink among her cleaning supplies. She was so relieved and so happy. But then she said, "Where is my house key? It should be in my purse." I said, "Please, Ellen, relax, take a deep breath, and look in your purse. It is probably in your purse." The key was in her purse.

On another day Ellen greeted me at her door in tears. She told me that she had just phoned her son and he had said, "Why do you keep calling me?" She told me she was hurt and lonely for her son. She said, "He never takes me out to dinner. He has forgotten that I used to take care of him. I don't ask much of him, and I realize that he is busy with his family. But I need to see him. I need to feel I have a family to care for me." Ellen sat in her favorite chair, and I sat on the floor next to her. I held her hand and looked directly into her eyes. Then I said, "Ellen, I'm happy that you told me about your feelings concerning your son. But you are wrong if you think your son does not love you. He does love you. He cares very much for you. Otherwise, I wouldn't be here with you today. He asked me to see you and to work with you on various activities. Your family does care about you, but sometimes they are so busy they cannot visit you." Ellen listened to me, stopped crying, and calmed down.

We played poker, and then we took a walk together. While we walked, Ellen talked about her husband whom she still missed even though he had died 14 years before. As we were walking back to her apartment, Ellen gave me her key and asked me to open her door—a break from custom. But when we reached her door, I gave her key back to her so she would open her door as usual. Nothing was said, but the giving and the returning of the key was a communication of trust. As we entered her apartment, Ellen said, "You know how to talk nice to me."

Build trust

This was an especially nice day. I took Ellen to the mall. She was so excited! On the way we stopped at a Dunkin Donuts shop. She had one doughnut and coffee. She refused a second doughnut, saying, "If I eat too much, I will not be able to walk. I have had enough. Thanks." Ellen thinks of consequences. Then Ellen said, "I like your company. But how do you know me? Who talked to you about me?" I told Ellen that her son had heard about me from friends and he had called me. After he talked to me, he introduced us. Ellen said, "But where is my son now?" I told her that he was in Florida on vacation. Ellen said, "It's okay; he can stay in Florida, but tell him I'm having a good time. What would I do without you?"

Ellen has become more and more relaxed. She seems to have gained more self-confidence and is happy to be able to make decisions, such as going to the mall, going out to eat, etc. It is essential that she not feel like a client in need of therapy. I trust that I am to her, a friend.

At the mall, Ellen enjoyed looking at the elegant, high fashion clothes. She has exquisite taste and comments knowingly about the various materials. She herself is always impeccably dressed. As we parted, Ellen gave me a hug and wished me luck.

Be A Friend

On another occasion, it was a down day for Ellen. She did not want to do anything. Her back hurt her. I noticed there was no toilet paper in her bathroom, and I told her so. She immediately stood up, and together we went downstairs to buy the needed paper. Then I said, "Since we are here, let's take a 10-minute walk." She agreed. Afterward, as she sat on her couch, she told me she had not seen her family recently. I reminded her that they were on vacation. She said, "Oh, okay."

She noticed an arrangement of fresh cut flowers in a vase and commented on their beautiful pink color. I asked Ellen if she saw any other color among the flowers. There were yellow, pink, and red flowers in the arrangement. Ellen said, "No, that's all." I said, "Ellen, I see some yellow flowers." Ellen said, "No, no, they are not pretty." It seems Ellen does not acknowledge the presence of what she does not like. I was surprised Ellen seems to dislike yellow.

Expressing independence

The other day I asked Ellen if she could play poker. She said she could, and I told her that I had always wanted to learn to play poker, but had never learned. I asked Ellen if she would teach me. Ellen seemed happy to do so. For a while she told me, step-by-step, what to do. But after a while, she became irritated at my incompetence and said, "I don't want to play because you don't know how. Forget it!" But Ellen was happy. She could play poker, and I couldn't.

Ellen and I were working on spelling puzzles when her daughter came in to visit her. When Ellen accepted a stick of gum from me, her daughter said, "Mother, you shouldn't have gum in your mouth. You know that you will forget you have the gum in your mouth and will end up swallowing it." Ellen retorted, "Why do you talk to me like that? You treat me with no respect. I would never swallow the gum. What's wrong with you?"

Resents authority

Then Ellen's daughter told her to take off her coat because the room was warm. Ellen responded, "No. I don't want to take my coat off. Why don't you take your coat off if you think it's hot in the room? Don't tell me what to do." An hour passed during which time Ellen and I continued with our usual activities. No word passed between mother and daughter. Ellen's daughter left.

It was lunchtime and Ellen insisted that she share her lunch with me. I told her I had a late breakfast and could not eat a thing. Ellen was firm, insisting that I must eat, at least, her salad. Seeing that my refusal was upsetting her, I said I would take the salad home with me. Ellen immediately relaxed, smiled, and said, "Okay."

Familiar things & places

I took Ellen to Sears. She remembered being there the week before. She liked and disliked the same dresses she did on the last visit. Later, Ellen wanted to go to an Espresso Shop. But this time she insisted on treating me because she remembered I had treated her last week. While we enjoyed our coffee, Ellen talked about her earlier life. She told me she and her husband had owned a big house and a clothing store where both she and her husband had worked hard together. I said that many people work hard to make money but still cannot earn enough money to buy a house. Ellen had no sympathy for such people and said, "Those people do not want to work, they just like money."

Limit the choices

One day, Ellen had difficulty dressing herself. Usually, she dresses in well-coordinated outfits. This day, however, she wore a hodgepodge outfit of mixed pieces. Sensing that Ellen was not satisfied with her appearance, I offered to help her find a blouse to match her pants. Ellen wanted no help and said she would help herself. She looked at herself in her closet mirror and selected a blue blouse to match her blue pants. But after putting on the blue blouse, she put on a pair of mauve-colored pants. She had overlooked the blue pants she had intended to wear. No sooner had she finished dressing herself in the blue blouse and mauve pants, she said, "Something is wrong here, but I don't know what it is." I said, "I will be happy to help you. Let's look for a blouse that matches your pants." With her consent, I offered her two choices. Finally, after changing her clothes several times, Ellen selected a pair of blue pants to match her blue blouse.

On another day, Ellen was not in her usual, good mood. Instead, she greeted me with a complaint. Her back hurt again. She responded to my greeting by telling me she wanted me to leave at once. She explained she was expecting company and asked that I please leave. I said that her plans were fine with me but her son wanted me to talk with her. Ellen said, "It does not matter what my son says." Not wanting to leave her in what I thought was a sad state; I offered to help her if she would tell me what was bothering her. She said, "No, thanks. I will tell you later. I just want you to leave, please. Come see me tomorrow." I said, "Okay," and I left her.

I went to the dining room and waited. Ellen usually does not stay long in her room but walks freely throughout the nursing home. One-half hour passed, and Ellen found me in the dining room. She said, "What are you doing here?" When I said I was waiting for her, she responded with, "Okay, let's go for a walk." After our walk, Ellen sat on a couch and said, "This place is exactly like the place I live in. Look, this chair is exactly like the chair in my place where I live." I said, "Ellen, this is the place where you live now." Ellen answered, "No, no! What's wrong with you? I moved yesterday from the place I used to live in because I didn't like it. I like this place better." I told her again that she was still living in the place she had been living in for quite some time. But she continued to insist she was living in a new place. Suddenly she said, "Look! You see that lady over there? She looks exactly like the lady I knew in the other place. Look! Even the flowers are the same as the ones in the other place."

Where am I?

Ellen was becoming quite agitated over what she seemed to perceive as being in a place identical to, but not in reality the same as her previous residence. To distract her, I gave her a small, soft ball to squeeze. This tactic seemed to work. Ellen grew calm. I suggested that we go to lunch, and she agreed. But after seating herself at her usual place, Ellen said, "God. I don't understand what is going on here. This chair and this table are exactly like the ones in the other place. Oh, look, look! I know all these people. They must have moved from the other place. They like it here better."

I looked straight into her eyes and said, "Ellen, you didn't move from your place. That is why all the people you see are familiar to you. You are sitting on the same chair and at the same table as you have been at ever since I started visiting you." Ellen replied, "Okay. I see. I thought I moved from here." I asked, "You don't mind living here, do you?" Ellen said, "No. It's okay with me. Anyway, I like it here." We dropped the subject, and Ellen had a good lunch. I believe that Ellen had the impression she was in a different home because she had encountered many unfamiliar faces at an open house party held at the nursing home the evening before.

Later, Ellen was in a good mood. She did not talk again about having moved, but said she felt childish when she had to write sentences. I told her writing sentences was good for the mind. She asked, "Why?" and said that it was hard to think of sentences. I explained that writing sentences would help keep her mind strong and writing was like taking a good vitamin. Ellen said "It is?" Then she started to write and also was very cooperative in playing memory games I had brought.

Just like a Vitamin

My next visit with Ellen found her beautifully dressed, in good spirits, and ready for an outing. She greeted me self-confidently. We conversed as good friends, each of us listening attentively to the other and asking questions from time to time. Ellen asked the same questions over and over, but I answered them as though she had never asked them before. Because Ellen seems so happy when she talks, I encourage her, and my reward is a more self-confident, happy Ellen.

After our walk, as we were returning to Ellen's apartment, Ellen greeted a fellow resident. Still in a happy mood, Ellen said to the resident, "Hello, it's good to see you." The resident glumly answered, "Thank you." Ellen continued, "Where did you come from? How did you get here?" The other resident did not respond. Ellen tried over and over to get the other resident to talk to her but couldn't get a response. Finally, Ellen asked me, "What's wrong with her? Why won't she talk to me?" I told Ellen that the woman had a hearing problem and she would have to excuse her. Ellen said, "Oh, okay. I feel sorry for her. She is a nice lady." Possibly, the other woman had no trouble hearing, but didn't understand the question. If Ellen had thought that the other resident just did not want to talk to her, her feelings may have been hurt and her happy mood destroyed.

Ellen asked me whether she had moved because everything she was seeing seemed new to her—the people were strangers, and the furniture was different. She said she did not want to be among strange people and wanted to go back to the place where she used to live. She said she wanted to be with the people she knew and to live in the place she knew.

Ride to the Rescue

She said she knew how to get to the beauty shop from the place where she used to live, but not from this place. Ellen strongly believed she was in a new nursing home and was tense and anxious about being in this "new" home—which, of course, was the same home she had been in for quite some time.

I decided to try to relieve her anxiety by suggesting we visit the home where she used to live. I then drove her to the mall and back home again. Her husband's picture was on her dresser, and I called her attention to it, asking, "Whose picture is that?" Ellen picked up the picture, looked at it, and said, "This is my husband. He died a long time ago. I wish he were still alive. The good people die early."

I told Ellen that she was now in the place she had lived in before. I asked her to look around. Her husband's picture was there and so were the people she had lived with before. Ellen looked around and said, "Yes, I feel I'm home. I know all these people, and everything is familiar. The other place was not good. It had bad food." When I took her to the dining room for lunch, she said, "Oh, I love the food here. It's better than the food in the other place."

One day, as I was approaching Ellen's apartment, I saw her leaving. I told her I had come to visit her and asked her where she was going. She said, "I'm bored. I don't know what is wrong with me. I want to go home." In her hand, she clutched her husband's picture. I asked her to come with me, and she said, "Why should I go with you?" I told her that I had something for her—her favorite fruit. Ellen asked, "What?" I told her black grapes.

Favorite fruits work

While following me back to her apartment, Ellen asked, "How do you know that I like grapes?" I told her I remembered that she had mentioned liking grapes and, because she was special to me, I had brought her some grapes. After we arrived at Ellen's apartment, I washed the grapes for her, and she enjoyed eating them.

Later I took her for a ride, and Ellen told me she was lonely. Her daughter and son were both away, and her husband was dead. I reminded her that her son had visited yesterday. Ellen reacted in a very agitated manner, saying, "What are you talking about? No, he was not here. He is in Florida." I told her I was sorry. Someone had told me that her son had visited with her yesterday, but she evidently was mistaken. After that, Ellen calmed down. After a few minutes, I asked Ellen if she had been able to keep her doctor's appointment yesterday. She said, "Yes." I said, "Oh, good. Who drove you to the doctor's office?" Ellen answered, "My son." I said, "Your son?" She said, "Yes." I said, "Oh, your son is back from Florida?" She said, "Yes." I said, "You see, your son comes almost every day to see you." Ellen said, "Oh, okay. You are right. My son is good to me." Ellen gradually started feeling better, and I bought her ice cream she liked. She even seemed happy as she ate her ice cream.

More Payback

On our ride back to her apartment, Ellen perked up. She told me, "I feel much better now. I really do. I can feel the difference, you know. Amira, God bless you. You make the difference. I feel like you are one of my daughters."

When we arrived at the nursing home, it was lunch time. Ellen said she was not hungry. I asked her if she would eat her lunch if I stayed with her. She said, "Yes," so I stayed with her, and she ate all her lunch.

On this day, as usual, Ellen asked where her son was. She told me she missed him and her daughter, who were both away. Her son visits her almost every day, but Ellen does not remember many of his visits.

Ellen told me she had no money in her purse. She then called her son at his office, forgetting she had called him earlier. Ellen was definitely acting more agitated than usual. She seemed to be on the verge of panic. I had never seen her in such a state.

As she sat next to the telephone crying, I asked her why she was so upset. She said, "I tried to call my son to talk to him, but he told me that I had just called him. I know that I did not call him before." I said, "Ellen, if your son said you called him earlier, he must be right." Ellen became upset with me.

I explained to her that when she calls her son, her calls are registered on his machine and she might have pressed the redial key by mistake. She said, "Okay, maybe that is possible. Now I want to call him because I need to talk to him." I said, "Ellen, your son is not in his office. Call him later." But she said, "I believe that my son went away without telling me. I need to know why. Because when he goes on a trip, I will be out on the street. I'm afraid he'll leave me with no money in my purse. I can't go anywhere without money."

Removing Roadblocks

Ellen was crying and said, "Let me call my son," and she did. His secretary told Ellen he was not in his office; he was on the road. The secretary told

Ellen she would tell her boss that his mother had called him. Ellen hung up the phone but kept saying she needed to see her son. She seemed on the verge of a panic attack when I had an idea. "Ellen, I have some money for you from your son." Ellen looked wide-eyed at me, smiled, and said, "Really, really? He gave you money for me?" I assured her he had, and I gave her some money to she put in her purse.

Soon Ellen seemed quite happy, and she willingly went for a walk with me. We participated in various recreational games, and she talked about her earlier life. After two weeks of wondering how to help cheer Ellen up, I had stumbled on her problem. She was afraid and insecure because she had no money in her purse—and no son readily available to reassure her. Now, with money in her purse, she relaxed, secure in the knowledge that she had money of her own.

Family visits are very important

When I arrived at Ellen's apartment one day, she was happily talking on the phone to her daughter. Excitedly, she told me that her daughter was coming to visit her. She did not want to leave her room because she was afraid she would miss her daughter. Ellen was so excited she seemed almost panicky. I told her to breathe slowly and take deep breaths, which she did. I convinced Ellen that her daughter would be coming into the lobby and she would be able to meet her there. Ellen said she did not want to go any place. She only wanted to wait for her daughter. So, she selected a chair in the lobby facing the entrance door and sat down to wait for her daughter.

I offered Ellen a newspaper to read while she waited, but she refused to take it, saying, "No. I don't feel like reading. All I want is wait for my daughter to come." After a while, I asked her if she would help me wind yarn on a spool. She said, "Okay," and began winding the yarn. After a few minutes, Ellen asked, "Do you know what time my daughter is coming?" I told her that her daughter would be there by evening. Ellen asked, "Is that what she said?" and I said, "Yes." Ellen said, "Oh, I have plenty of time to do things." Then I proposed we play poker, and Ellen agreed. We played poker and other games, but from time to time Ellen would ask me when her daughter would be coming. Finally, she said, "Yeah, my daughter never rushes to see me. She does not know how much I miss her." The next day I asked Ellen if her daughter had visited her the evening before. She smiled and said, "Yes, she visited me." Ellen was calm and more alert than usual. She seemed to be happy, remembering her daughter's visit.

Go with the flow

I had been phoning Ellen from time to time between visits. When she answered the telephone, she would ask who I am. I would tell her my name and say, "Ellen, you know me. I'm the friend who comes to visit you." Then she would laugh and say, "Yes, I recognize your voice. You are the lady with the last name that is hard to pronounce." I would say, "That is right, but what is my first name?" (I tell them it's Amy because it is easier to pronounce than Amira.) Ellen says, "I forget," and I ask, "How do you pronounce A-M-Y?" Then Ellen says, "Oh, oh, Amy. Now I remember your name." Ellen likes to talk on the phone with me. She tells me what bothers her and what makes her happy. Today she said, "I feel good when you call me. You must care about me. You are a nice lady." It seems that my calls to Ellen and to my other clients are as important to them as my visits. If they know that I am not being paid to telephone them, it reinforces their feelings of being liked and cared for.

If you can't visit—call instead

Today Ellen was not in a good mood. She asked me to help her telephone her sister. I reminded Ellen that her sister had died years earlier, but I did not know if she had two sisters. Ellen said, "No. I have only one sister. She did not die. What is wrong with you?" I said, "Okay, I'm sorry." Ellen continued, "My sister is looking after me. My son wants me, and my daughter wants me, too. Every one of my family needs me. Why don't you understand?"

I said, "Okay, let's call your sister. What is your sister's name?" She said, "Ellen," and handed me a card. I looked at the card and said, "Ellen, this card that you have given me has your name and your telephone number on it. How can I call your sister?" Ellen answered, "No. Call her now. My sister's name is Ellen, too. This is her telephone number."

Amira C. Tame, A.C.C.

I dialed Ellen's telephone and handed Ellen the telephone so she could listen. Ellen said, "Oh, God, nobody is home. Damn it! My sister just called me a few minutes ago. Where did she go?" She became very agitated. Hoping to forestall panic, I suggested, "Let's go downstairs. Maybe your sister is waiting for you there." Relaxing a little, Ellen said, "Okay, let's go."

Holidays are uplifting

On the way downstairs, I said, "Ellen, Mother's Day is coming soon." Smiling slightly, she said, "Oh, yes." I asked which Mother's Days she remembered. Ellen said, "Oh, I got a lot of presents, and my family came to see me and took me out." I said, "Right. On Mother's Day every one of your family is coming to see you, and you will be treated like a very special lady." I continued a conversation about Mother's Day, and Ellen seemed to relax, letting a bit of happiness surface into a slight smile. By the time we got downstairs, Ellen had forgotten all she had been saying about her sister. She asked, "What are we supposed to do here?" I told her she needed to do her daily walking exercise, and she calmly replied, "Oh, yes." Ellen talked about how happy she was in her apartment.

Mood vs. Memory

Later, when I called her in the evening, Ellen remembered me as the lady who takes care of her. She said, "How nice that you called me. You make me feel good." Ellen talked for some time about her feelings before she said, "Good-bye," and hung up.

Three days after Mother's Day, Ellen is still glowing from the love and attention she received from her family on that day. Her smiling eyes radiate contentment, and she says she wishes that every day were Mother's Day, so she could be with her children and her grandchildren.

Usually, I ask Ellen to join me for a walk, but today, in her upbeat mood, Ellen asked *me*. While we were walking, Ellen saw a family of parents and children. She selected a seat from where she could watch them and said, "Look at those kids. Aren't they cute?" She was totally absorbed in watching them and ignored my attempts to talk with her. When she was ready to leave, Ellen joined me in a word game which she seemed to enjoy.

Build on positive feelings

Ordinarily, her blinds are kept closed against the bright morning sunlight; however, the housekeeper had left them open. Ellen could see the beautiful, green, leaf laden trees, shrubs, and lawn and said, "Oh, my gosh! How did you get here? You are very nice to come," and she gave me a hug. I said, "Ellen, I don't live far from here." Ellen said, "What do you mean? I know that you live in a cold place, and I've come to Florida. Don't you see outside how nice and green it is? I like Florida better than that place I used to live in."

I told Ellen she was right, but we were still living in Michigan, and it was now warm and sunny because it was Springtime. I said, "Sometimes Michigan has warm, nice days just like Florida." Ellen protested, saying, "What are you talking about? No, I am in Florida on vacation. I want to stay here. It's nice here." I asked her if she would like to go outside for a walk. She did. While we were leaving the building, Ellen saw some of the residents and said, "Some of the people here look like people I know." I asked her why she liked Florida, and she said, "Because Florida is nice and warm and green." I said, "Michigan's weather today looks like Florida's warm weather."

Ellen has improved considerably. Obviously suffering from a loss of self-esteem and exhibiting antisocial behavior, Ellen has become an outgoing, happy person. I intend to do all that I can to help Ellen improve more and more.

Alice

Alice and I play word games together. When she encounters a word she cannot spell, rather than say she can't spell it, she says, "I have done enough. I don't want to play anymore." So, rather than spell words, we name things. When Alice looks at an object, she can name it; but she has a difficult time remembering things that are out of sight. She has a visual type personality, and this trait is very important when deciding what techniques to utilize.

Amira C. Tame, A.C.C.

Martha

Martha seemed to be in an advanced stage of Alzheimer's disease. When I first spoke to her, she ignored me. So, I spoke loudly to her. She still ignored me. Then I took her hand, bent down, and looked into her eyes. Speaking softly, I said, "Martha." Martha then looked at me as though waiting to hear what I was going to say. I said, "Martha, I am going to sing a song, and I would like you to sing with me. You do?" Martha sang with me. She didn't like being shouted at. So, she tunes out shouters. Martha's face is peaceful. She never displays anger or hostility. I sense that she receives, a lot of love and care from her family.

On this day, Martha is in a bad mood. She has never wanted to participate in any activity, but she usually will sing with me. Today, however, she only makes her usual sound, "Eh, eh, eh . . ." When I spoke to her, she looked at me angrily and said loudly, "No. No." Seeing that she was angry and highly agitated, I remained quiet. I sat close to her, took her hand, and looked questioningly into her eyes. But she said nothing. Eventually, Martha tried to say something, but I did not understand her. Fifteen minutes passed. Martha became quiet. Five more minutes passed in silence. Then Martha hit my hand and said, "Woo!" She smiled at me and I said, "Martha, you scared me." Martha said, "I did? I woke you up!" I was amazed because Martha has rarely spoken. After that, Martha seemed calm and relaxed. So, I asked her if she would pick up the big beads and put them in the tray. To my surprise, she did. She worked with beads and string for a while, seemingly in a good mood, and was very cooperative. My purpose was to let Martha know that she was free to do what she wanted to do and was in no way obligated to do anything I wanted her to do. I think Martha realized that she was respected and her wishes were important.

Go with the flow

Martha had difficulty holding a ball or anything else. I tried to interest her in stringing beads, but she would not touch the beads or the string. She wanted to only watch me while she made her usual noise, "Eh, eh, eh . . ." Suddenly she became quiet. Her eyes were closed. I was concerned and said, "Martha, Martha, are you okay?" Martha opened her eyes, looked at me, and said, "Yes. I'm okay. I just fell asleep. The beads moving across the string put me to sleep. "Eh, eh, eh." I was surprised that watching the stringing of the beads made her fall asleep. I didn't quite believe it, but twice again I strung beads, and twice again Martha fell asleep. Martha has come a long way since I first started seeing her just a few weeks ago.

From absolutely refusing to use her hands in any way, Martha has now progressed to the point where she will touch things she is looking at. She will touch a magazine but will not turn its pages. Martha likes to listen to classical music and watch me do various things, but her responses are mainly, "Eh, eh, eh . . ." Martha now seems to be much more aware of what is happening around her than when I originally met her.

Andrea

Andrea greeted my "Good morning!" with, "Oh, yes. What?" I said, "Andrea, it's a beautiful day, and the sun is shining. It's a good day to smile." She said, "What for?" I asked if something was bothering her. Andrea said, "I don't know. I'm unhappy with myself," and she started to cry.

I looked directly into Andrea's eyes and said, "Andrea, we all have good days, and we all have bad days, but that does not mean we are not okay. You are probably having a bad day, but you are okay." Andrea said, "Do you think so?" I assured her I did and she stopped crying. I asked her if she would like to go for a ride, and she said, "Okay." She went to her room to get dressed and promptly started to swear because she couldn't find her panty hose. I found them for her, under her bed. Andrea remembered my car and went directly to it. It is a black car. Andrea said she liked my car because it was big and white. I suggested that my car might not be white but black. "No," Andrea insisted, "Your car is white." I told Andrea I liked white cars too.

At the mall, Andrea looked at cosmetics and jewelry, comparing prices. She seemed relaxed and talked about things that interested her. I asked her if she felt better or was she still upset. Andrea said, "I was not upset or sad." Andrea had forgotten that she had been in a bad mood earlier.

Sometimes black is white

When we returned to Andrea's apartment, I asked her what color my car was. She said, "Black." I asked her if she had seen me driving a white car, and she answered, "You always drive a black car. What's wrong with you?"

Ramona

Ramona lives in a nursing home. One day she was playing with a boy baby doll and said, "I like my baby. He just looks at me and never talks back to me." I asked if he had a name. Ramona said, "No, but it doesn't matter because he doesn't talk." She would loan her doll to other patients and her friends. She told me that her doll made her friends happy because he always smiled. The baby-boy doll did seem to relax the women and bring smiles to their faces.

I brought Ramona a basket of artificial flowers, and she set about happily rearranging them in the basket. I asked her what her favorite color was, and she said she did not know. Then I asked her which color she liked best of all. Ramona seemed reluctant to choose from among so many colors. I picked up one flower and asked, "Do you like this color?" Ramona said, "I don't know." Then I picked up a blue flower and a yellow one and asked, "Ramona, which flower do you like, the blue or the yellow flower?" She pointed to the yellow flower and I put the blue flower away.

Favorites by observation

I picked a pink flower and asked, "Ramona, which flower do you like, the yellow flower or the pink flower?" Ramona again pointed to the yellow flower. I did this repeatedly with each of the variously-colored flowers. Eventually, I learned that Ramona's favorite colors were yellow and pink. It seems that Ramona could decide between one of two colors, but she could not make a selection if she had more than two colors to consider. After this little experiment, Ramona was smiling and relaxed. She now knew her favorite color was yellow and pink was next.

Jane

While Jane and I were working on a puzzle, her son came to visit her. Jane asked him if he had come yesterday, and he said he had. Jane said, "I don't remember that you came here." "Mom," her son said, "you know that your mind is going blank." Jane became silent. It was a blow from her beloved son to her self-esteem.

OOPS!
Didn't Check the Survey Form

One day I brought my two parakeets with me to Jane's apartment. After our usual greeting, I said, "Guess what, Jane? You have a visitor. Guess who?" Jane said, "Who?" "Look in the box," I said, "and you will know." Jane looked in the box and, upon seeing the parakeets, said in an angry voice, "What is this? I don't like birds at all. Who told you to bring birds to my apartment? Get them out right now! I'm not crazy about birds." I apologized, saying, "I didn't mean to upset you," and I put the birds out in the hallway. Jane wouldn't talk for quite a while after that. Finally, I asked Jane if she would like to go for a walk with me. She agreed. While we walked, I sang the song, "Let Me Call You Sweetheart," and Jane sang along with me. Soon Jane tired of walking and said she wanted to sit down.

I asked Jane to write a sentence for me and she said, "Like what?" I told her anything she could think of and added that I needed six sentences from her. Jane wrote the following:

When Jane gave me her six sentences, I said, "Jane, you wrote all six sentences the same. Write something different." Jane replied, "What are you talking about? I wrote down different hours in my sentences.

I can't think of anything else." As far as she was concerned, it met the requirement. I agreed.

Sally and Sarah

I have two new residents who are sisters and have been very close all of their lives. Although they live in the same nursing home, each has her own room. Sally and Sarah visit one another several times a day. Sarah's daughter asked me to work with Sarah one-on-one without Sally in the room. But Sarah was opposed to this. She told me she had done enough activities in her life, and now all she wanted to do was relax and enjoy time with her sister. Sarah said she would do nothing without her sister. So, rather than waste her time and mine, I went to her sister's room and brought Sally to Sarah. Sally wanted to know what I was doing in Sarah's room. I told her I was there as a friend, and we could all go out together and we could play games.

Activities can be fun

Sally and Sarah talked to each other and decided it would be okay to play with the balloon. After batting the balloon back and forth for a while, Sarah said, "I'm happy to be your friend." And Sally added, "I'm happy to be your friend, too."

After tiring of the balloon, Sarah and Sally played with a word puzzle where the object is to spell simple words. But, after agreeing to play, Sarah said, "I feel dumb. I'm not smart anymore in my old age." And Sally said, "I don't feel smart anymore either." I pointed out the words they had spelled correctly and told them they had done well. Then I said, "Don't you feel proud of yourselves?" Each one said she did. Then Sarah gave me a hug and said, "I haven't had so much fun in a long time."

Job to the Rescue

Sarah greeted me with a smile. Seeing my briefcase (in which I carry my activity supplies), she asked what I was selling today. I told her I did not have anything to sell but I did have some puzzle games. When I suggested she and I put some puzzles together, Sarah said, "Oh, good." As she worked on the puzzles, she talked about how much she missed her daughters.

She also talked about the way things used to be—the work she used to do when she was a "telephone operator" and how poor she was during World War II.

This day's routine with Sally was the same as it usually is. We walked, and her smiling countenance betrayed no turmoil or discontent. Her daily routine is broken once a week by a trip to the beauty salon where Sally has her hair washed, set, and styled.

On another day, Sally seemed to be in a bad mood. She also appeared to be depressed. She did not want to walk. She did not want to talk. She only wanted to watch television. I asked Sally if I could turn off the TV. She said, "Okay." Because Sally usually likes to talk about the job she used to have, I asked her about her job. Sally then talked at some length about her job selling clothes. After talking for most of the two-hour session, Sally seemed to perk up and said that she would like to go for a walk. So, we walked and after that, we played word games.

Sally's seemingly happy mood did not last long for she evidently took a dislike toward a new resident who was sitting at the lunch table. Sally left the table saying, "I'm not hungry. I have to go to my room." But then she asked the aide to take her lunch to her room, explaining to me that she couldn't like that "guest lady." Then she told me she did not know why, but she hated her. Sally seemed to enjoy her lunch in her room and asked me to join her, which, after first declining and upon her insistence, I did. While we ate lunch together, Sally seemed to relax and regain her contented mood.

When I visited Sarah, I found her daughter with her. The nursing home had called Sarah's daughter to come because she had been "misbehaving." Her daughter had managed to calm Sarah, but she was still in quite a bad mood. After her daughter left, I asked her about the job she used to have. She loved to talk about the experiences she had when she was an operator at the telephone company, and she happily recounted some of those experiences.

Nobody's perfect

After some time, I asked Sarah if she would help me arrange flowers in a basket. She likes to make beautiful floral arrangements, so she took

Amira C. Tame, A.C.C.

over the job. Later, we played a spelling game together, but she became frustrated and angry when she could not remember how to spell a certain word. Although I told her it was okay to make mistakes and that everyone makes mistakes, she did not agree. I pretended I was mixed up and had forgotten how to spell a simple word. Sarah said, "See, you are mixed up, too!" I said, "Nobody is perfect. We all make mistakes." Hearing this admission seemed to calm Sarah.

After the spelling game, I asked Sarah to join me in "arm exercises," e.g., batting a balloon back and forth. She agreed. Once before I had asked her to "play balloon" with me and she had refused, saying that was kids' play and she was not a kid. We did these exercises for a while for "our health." Suddenly, Sarah abruptly told me to go home, saying, she had a headache. I said, "No problem. I'll go. I understand you don't feel well." It was time for me to go anyway. To hasten me on my way, Sarah helped me put my activity supplies in my briefcase.

It was my day with Sarah. She always tells me that she has had enough activity in her life and all she wants to do now is relax. But I know Sarah will arrange flowers in a basket and will readily talk about her past. Today she even folded some towels, after first arranging her flowers. I asked Sarah if she liked surprises, and she said, "Yes."

I placed a bowl before her that I had filled with sand under which I had buried a quarter and a few pieces of old costume jewelry. I told Sarah to feel around in the bowl until she felt something and guess what it was. Sarah was able to guess what most of the items were, and she bubbled over with happiness when she pulled out an item and found that she had guessed right. Ordinarily, Sarah won't use her hands, but she will use them if she is having fun doing something. The next week when I met with Sarah, her sister Sally was visiting her. Sarah noticed the case in which I carry my activity supplies and asked, "What are you going to sell me today? I have no money to buy from you." I told Sarah I was not a sales person—I was her activity therapist, and she and I were going to work on some word games. She apologized and said, "I didn't remember you, but now I do."

I asked Sarah if she would help me peel some potatoes. She agreed, and we peeled potatoes while she talked about how she used to cook for her husband. Her curiosity aroused, Sarah asked what I was going to do with the potatoes. I told her that I was going to cook some potatoes when I got home and I thought she would help me.

Fear of being alone

Soon Sally said she was going back to her room because her daughter and her mother were coming to visit her. Objecting, Sarah said to Sally, "Your mother died a long time ago. What is wrong with you? Besides, I don't want you to leave me here alone." I reminded Sarah that she was not alone, that I was with her. But Sarah said, "I know you are going to leave after a little while, and I will be alone. I hate to be alone. I hate it. I hate it. I hate it. I'm afraid to be alone."

Sally told Sarah, "My family comes first. I can't stay with you all the time." The telephone rang. Sarah's daughter was calling. She told Sarah that she would be coming to visit her soon. Sarah told her daughter it would be nice if she would come over. But after she hung up, Sarah told me, "I hate it when my daughter tells me she is coming to see me and then doesn't show up. She just promises and doesn't come." I told Sarah that her daughter always visits her when she says she will. Sarah disagreed, saying, "No. I know my daughter, and I remember the times she did not show up. Do you think I am senile?"

Disappointment Hurts

Sarah waited and waited for her daughter to come, but her daughter did not come. After waiting quite a while for her daughter, Sarah grew agitated and said she did not feel like doing anything. Sarah told me she knew her daughter had lied to her several times and she no longer fully believed what her daughter told her. She asked me to telephone her daughter. I called Sarah's daughter after I got home and asked her if she was coming to visit her mother. Sarah's daughter told me that she was too busy to come and she had only told her mother she was going to visit her because she knew that her mother would not remember. I told Sarah's daughter what she had told me, emphasizing that she did remember her daughter's promises and the times her daughter did not keep her promises. I also told Sarah's daughter she was sad and disappointed because of those broken promises.

Later that evening, I called Sarah and asked her if she remembered me. She said, "Yes. You are the lady selling things." I said, "No. Sarah, I am your activities therapist." She said, "Oh, okay," and then she told me about some things that were bothering her. She seemed to enjoy talking on the telephone and told me, "How nice of you to call me. I feel good when I talk to you because I can get everything out of my system."

One day, Sarah greeted me at her door by stating, "I'm not ready to do any activities today. I'm supposed to go out with my daughter. She will be here any minute. I think you have come at the wrong time." I told Sarah that it would be nice for her to be with her daughter but her daughter would not be coming until after our activities session. Becoming visibly agitated, Sarah said, "I have waited for a long time for this opportunity to see my daughter." I said, "Okay, I'm leaving. I'll see you soon." I went to the waiting room for a short time, and while returning to see her again, I saw she was on her way to the waiting room. I said, "Hello, Sarah." She looked at me and said, "Sorry, you've come at the wrong time." I had thought she would have forgotten the earlier episode, but she had not. She was adamant. She would not participate in any activity and would only wait for her daughter. I telephoned Sarah's daughter, and she explained to me that she would be visiting her mother later in the afternoon. It was not yet mid-morning.

Later in the evening, I called Sarah and asked her whether she had enjoyed her visit that afternoon with her daughter. Sarah did not remember her daughter's visit, but she enjoyed talking to me on the telephone and said she was looking forward to seeing me again.

Janet

One resident, Janet, concerned me. She never spoke and never participated in any of the activities. My supervisor and the staff were not troubled by this because Janet had not spoken since she entered the nursing home. Everyone seemed to assume that Janet was simply antisocial.

One day, Janet approached the TLC Class and looked at me. I welcomed her with a smile and told her that we would all be very happy if she would join the team. Janet just stared at me. She did not smile. She did not speak.

Meanwhile, the residents were enjoying the cookies and coffee I had been serving, and I invited Janet to join us. She ate the cookies and glumly accepted the attention that I gave her.

Day-by-day Janet's interest grew in subtle ways. She would color part of a picture and impassively and silently accept praise for her work. Although Janet's attitude had greatly improved, she still did not overtly respond to anyone nor did she speak. She continued to irritate some of the residents by continually staring at them.

Evidently Janet was responding to me in a way that I could not see. I had been seeing gradual improvement in her participation for about three months when one morning I returned to the nursing home after a day off and found her looking for me. She came to me, hugged me and said, "I love you."

Amazed, I hurried to my supervisor's office and told everyone what Janet had said to me. They all were happy and surprised that Janet had spoken. They wanted to know how I had induced her to talk. Looking back, I think that I had just made Janet feel wanted and loved. Janet continued to improve her relationships with other residents and became an active participant in my activities.

My hopes and dreams of helping those suffering from Alzheimer's disease have come to fruition with the completion of this book. For many years I've been seeing improvements first hand and have felt the satisfaction of making a positive difference in the lives of your loved ones. I hope that using these therapeutic activities will be as rewarding for you and your loved ones as it is for me and my clients. It is difficult to find the words to describe the deep feelings that surfaced as I reached for remnants of memory to build upon. It is even more difficult to describe the euphoria I feel each time I see a smile on the face of someone who has had little to smile about. Imagine the comfort and satisfaction of seeing deteriorated relationships return to being productive and meaningful ones.

Amira C. Tame, A.C.C.

Appendix

ALABAMA

Alabama Commission on Aging
RSA Plaza, Suite 470
770 Washington Avenue
Montgomery, AL 36130-1851
(334) 242-5743 FAX: (334) 242 5594

ALASKA

Alaska Commission on Aging
Division of Senior Services
Department of Administration
P.O. Box110209
Juneau, AK 99811-0209
(907) 465-3250 FAX: (907) 465-4716

ARIZONA

Aging and Adult Administration
Department of Economic Security
1789 West Jefferson Street—#950A-2SW
Phoenix, AZ 85007
(602) 542-4446 FAX: (602) 542-6575

ARKANSAS

Division Aging and Adult Services
Arkansas Dept of Human Services
P.O. Box 1437, Slot 1412
1417 Donaghey Plaza South
Little Rock, AR 72203-1437
(501) 682-2441 FAX: (501) 682-8155

CALIFORNIA

California Department of Aging
1600 K Street
Sacramento, CA 95814
(916) 322-3887 FAX: (916) 324-4989

COLORADO

Aging and Adult Services
Department of Social Services
110-16th Street, Suite 200
Denver, CO 80202-4147
(303) 866-2800 FAX: (303) 866-2696

CONNECTICUT

Division of Elderly Services
25 Sigourney Street, 10th Floor
Hartford, CT 06106-5033
(800) 994-9422
FAX: (860) 424-4966

DELAWARE

*Delaware Division of Services for Aging
and Adults with Physical Disabilities*
Department of Health and Social Services
1901 North DuPont Highway
New Castle, DE 19720
(302) 577-4791 or (800) 223-9074
FAX: (302) 577-4793

DISTRICT OF COLUMBIA

District of Columbia Office on Aging
One Judiciary Square—9th Floor
441 Fourth Street, N.W., Suite 900—South
Washington, DC 20001
(202) 724-5622
FAX: (202) 724-4979

FLORIDA

Department of Elder Affairs
Building B—Suite 152
4040 Esplanade Way
Tallahassee, FL 32399-7000
(850) 414-2000
FAX: (850) 414-2004

GEORGIA

Division of Aging Services
Department of Human Resources
2 Peachtree Street NW, Suite 9-398
Atlanta, GA 30303-3142
(404) 657-5258
FAX: (404) 657-5285

HAWAII

Hawaii Executive Office on Aging
250 South Hotel Street, Suite 406
Honolulu, HI 96813-2831
(808) 586-0100 FAX: (808) 586-0185

IDAHO

Idaho Commission on Aging
3380 Americana Terrace, Suite 120
Boise, ID 83706
(208) 334-3833 FAX: (208) 334-3033

ILLINOIS

Illinois Department on Aging
421 East Capitol Avenue, Suite 100
Springfield, IL 62701-1789
(217) 785-2870 or (800) 252-8966
Chicago Office: (312) 814-2916
FAX: (217) 785-4477

INDIANA

Bureau of Aging and In-Home Services
Division of Disability, Aging and
Rehabilitative Services
Family and Social Services Administration
402 W. Washington Street, #W454
P.O. Box 7083
Indianapolis, IN 46207-7083
(317) 232-7020 FAX: (317) 232-7867

IOWA

Iowa Department of Elder Affairs
Clemens Building, 3rd Floor
200 Tenth Street, Suite 300
Des Moines, IA 50309-3609
(515) 281-5187 FAX: (515) 281-5187

KANSAS

Department on Aging
New England Building
503 S. Kansas Ave.
Topeka, KS 66603-3404
785-296-4986 or (800) 432-3535
FAX: 785-296-0256

KENTUCKY

Office of Aging Services
Cabinet for Families and Children
Commonwealth of Kentucky
275 East Main Street
Frankfort, KY 40621
(502) 564-6930 FAX: (502) 564-4595

LOUISIANA

Governor's Office of Elderly Affairs
P.O. Box 80374
Baton Rouge, LA 70898-0374
(225) 342-7100 FAX: (225) 342-7133

MAINE

Bureau of Elder and Adult Services
Department of Human Services
35 Anthony Avenue
State House—Station #11
Augusta, ME 04333
(207) 624-5335 or (800) 262-2232
FAX: (207) 624-5361

MARYLAND

Maryland Department of Aging
State Office Building, Room 1007
301 West Preston Street
Baltimore, MD 21201-2374
(800) AGE-DIAL FAX: (410) 333-7943

MASSACHUSETTS

Massachusetts Executive Office of Elder
Affairs
One Ashburton Place, 5th Floor
Boston, MA 02108
(617) 727-7750
FAX: (617) 727-9368

MICHIGAN

Michigan Office of Services to the Aging
611 W. Ottawa, N. Ottawa Tower, 3rd Floor
P.O. Box 30676
Lansing, MI 48909
(517) 373-8230
FAX: (517) 373-4092

MINNESOTA

Aging and Adult Services
444 Lafayette Road
St. Paul, MN 55155-3843
(651) 296-2544
FAX: (651) 296-7855

MISSISSIPPI

Division of Aging and Adult Services
750 N. State Street
Jackson, MS 39202
(601) 359-4929 or (800) 346-6347
FAX: (601) 359-4370

MISSOURI

Division of Aging
Department of Social Services
P.O. Box 1337
615 Howerton Court
Jefferson City, MO 65102-1337
(573) 751-3082 or (800) 235-5503
FAX: (573) 751-8687

MONTANA

Senior and Long Term Care Division
Department of Public Health & Human
Services
P.O. Box 4210
111 Sanders, Room 211
Helena, MT 59620
(406) 444-7788 or (800) 332-2272
FAX: (406) 444-7743

NEBRASKA

Department of Health and Human Services
Division on Aging
P.O. Box 95044
1343 M Street
Lincoln, NE 68509-5044
(402) 471-2307
FAX: (402) 471-4619

NEVADA

Nevada Division of Aging Services
Department of Human Resources
State Mail Room Complex
3416 Goni Road, Building D
Carson City, NV 89706
Phone: (775) 687-4210
Fax: (775) 687-4264

NEW HAMPSHIRE

Division of Elderly and Adult Services
State Office Park South
129 Pleasant Street, Brown Bldg. #1
Concord, NH 03301
(603) 271-4680
FAX: (603) 271-4643

NEW JERSEY

Department of Health and Senior Services
New Jersey Division of Senior Affairs
P.O Box 807
Trenton, New Jersey 08625-0807
(609) 588-3141 or (800) 792-8820
FAX: (609) 588-3601

NEW MEXICO

New Mexico Aging & Long-Term Services
Department
2550 Cerrillos Road
Santa Fe, NM 87505
(505) 476-4799 or
Toll free NM only—(866) 451-2901
Resource Center—(800) 432-2080

NEW YORK

New York State Office for The Aging
2 Empire State Plaza
Albany, NY 12223-1251
(518) 474-5731 or (800) 342-9871
FAX: (518) 474-0608

NORTH CAROLINA

Department of Health and Human Services Division of Aging
2101 Mail Service Center
Raleigh, NC 27699-2101
(919) 733-3983
FAX: (919) 733-0443

NORTH DAKOTA

Department of Human Services Aging Services Division
600 South 2nd Street, Suite 1C
Bismarck, ND 58504
(701) 328-8910
FAX: (701) 328-8989

OHIO

Ohio Department of Aging
50 West Broad Street—9th Floor
Columbus, OH 43215-5928
(614) 466-5500
FAX: (614) 466-5741

OKLAHOMA

Aging Services Division
Department of Human Services
P.O. Box 25352
312 N.E. 28th Street
Oklahoma City, OK 73125
(405) 521-2281 or 521-2327
FAX: (405) 521-2086

OREGON

Department of Human Services—Seniors
500 Summer Street, N.E., 2nd Floor
Salem, OR 97310-1015
(503) 945-5811
FAX: (503) 373-7823

PENNSYLVANIA

Pennsylvania Department of Aging
Commonwealth of Pennsylvania
555 Walnut Street, 5th floor
Harrisburg, PA 17101-1919
(717) 783-1550
FAX: (717) 772-3382

RHODE ISLAND

Department of Elderly Affairs
160 Pine Street
Providence, RI 02903-3708
(401) 222-2858
FAX: (401) 222-1490

SOUTH CAROLINA

Office of Senior and Long Term Care Services
Department of Health and Human Services
P.O. Box 8206
Columbia, SC 29202-8206
(803) 898-2501
FAX: (803) 898-4515

SOUTH DAKOTA

Office of Adult Services and Aging
Richard F. Kneip Building
700 Governors Drive
Pierre, SD 57501-2291
(605) 773-3656
FAX: (605) 773-6834

TENNESSEE

Commission on Aging
Andrew Jackson Building. 9th floor,
500 Deaderick Street,
Nashville, Tennessee 37243-0860
(615) 741-2056
FAX: (615) 741-3309

TEXAS

Texas Department on Aging
4900 North Lamar, 4th Floor
Austin, TX 78751-2316
(512) 424-6840
FAX: (512) 424-6890

UTAH

Division of Aging & Adult Services
Box 45500
120 North 200 West
Salt Lake City, UT 84145-0500
(801) 538-3910
FAX: (801) 538-4395

VERMONT

Vermont Department of Aging and Disabilities
Waterbury Complex
103 South Main Street
Waterbury, VT 05671-2301
(802) 241-2400
FAX: (802) 241-2325

VIRGINIA

Virginia Department for the Aging
1600 Forest Avenue, Suite 102
Richmond, VA 23229
(804) 662-9333 or (800) 662-9354
FAX: (804) 662-9354

WASHINGTON

Aging and Adult Services Administration
Department of Social & Health Services
P.O. Box 45050
Olympia, WA 98504-5050
(360) 493-2500 FAX: (360) 438-8633

WEST VIRGINIA

West Virginia Bureau of Senior Services
1900 Kanawha Boulevard East
Charleston, WV 25305
(877) 987-4463 FAX: (304) 558-5609

WISCONSIN

Department of Health and Family Services
P.O. Box 7851
Madison, WI 53707
(608) 266-1865
FAX: (608) 267-3203

WYOMING

Office on Aging
Department of Health
6101 Yellowstone Road, Room 259B
Cheyenne, WY 82002
(307) 777-7996 or (800) 442-2766
FAX: (307) 777-5340

Dementia and Caregiving Selected National/State Resources

Alzheimer's Disease Education & Referral (ADEAR) Center
A service of the National Institute on Aging PO Box 8250, Silver Spring, MD 20907-8250 Phone: (800) 438-4380
This information clearinghouse provides information to caregivers and practitioners. The center publishes a newsletter and offers a catalog of inexpensive audio/visual materials for training.

Benjamin B. Green-Field National Alzheimer's Library and Resource Center
(Alzheimer's Association)
919 North Michigan Avenue, Suite 1000
Chicago IL 60611-1676
Phone: (312) 335-9602
Fax: (312) 335-0214
E-mail: greenfld@alz.org
Web Site: (Alzheimer's Association page)
http://www.alz.org/assoc/contact.html
The center has developed 24 bibliographies on frequently requested subjects, including behavioral symptoms, family caregiver stress and respite services.

Duke Family Support Program
Center for the Study of Aging and Human Development
Box 3600 Duke University Medical Center
Durham, NC 27710
Phone: (919) 660-7510
Web Site: under construction
This program offers a number of inexpensive print and audio/visual materials on dementia and caregiving.

Family Caregiver Alliance
425 Bush Street, suite 500
San Francisco, CA 94108
Phone: (415) 434-3388
Web Site: http://www.caregiver.org
clearinghouse.

Amira C. Tame, A.C.C.

National Alzheimer's Association SAFE RETURN Program
This is the only national program developed to help people who are at risk for wandering. The program helps identify, locate and return individuals who are memory impaired due to Alzheimer's disease or a related disorder. For more information regarding the **SAFE RETURN PROGRAM,** contact your local Alzheimer's Association Chapter or call **1-800-272-3900.**

Further information:
American Academy of Neurology
1080 Montreal Avenue
St. Paul, MN 55116-2325
(612) 695-1940
Fax (612) 695-2791
Web site: http://www.aan.com

Alzheimer's Disease Education and Referral Center
PO Box 8250
Silver Spring, MD 20907-8250
(800) 438-4380
Fax: (301) 495-3334
E-mail: adear@alzheimers.org
Web site: http://www.alzheimers.org/adear

The Alzheimer's Foundation
8177 South Harvard
M/C—114
Tulsa, OK 74137
(918) 481-6031

State Human Service Agency Information

Alabama

Agency: Alabama Department of Human Resources

Public Information Number: (334) 242-1850
Agency: Alabama Medicaid Agency
Public Information Number: (334) 242-5610

Alaska

Agency: Alaska Department of Health and Social Services
Public Information Number: (907) 465-3030

Arizona

Agency: Arizona Department of Economic Security
Public Information Number: (602) 542-4296
Agency: Arizona Health Care Cost Containment System
Public Information Number: (602) 417-4424

Arkansas

Agency: Arkansas Department of Human Services
Public Information Number: (501) 682-8650

California

Agency: California Health and Human Services Agency
Public Information Number: (916) 654-3454

Colorado

Agency: Colorado Department of Health Care Policy and Financing
Public Information Number: (303) 866-2868
Agency: Colorado Department of Human Services
Public Information Number: (303) 866-5822

Connecticut

Agency: Connecticut Department of Children and Families
Public Information Number: (860) 550-6305
Agency: Connecticut Department of Social Services
Public Information Number: (860) 424-5012

Delaware

Agency: Delaware Health and Social Services
Public Information Number: (302) 255-9037
Agency: Delaware Department of Services for Children, Youth, and Their Families
Public Information Number: (302) 633-2501
District of Columbia
Agency: D.C. Department of Health
Public Information Number: (202) 442-9195
Agency: D.C. Department of Human Services
Public Information Number: (202) 279-6127

Florida

Agency: Florida Agency for Health Care Administration
Public Information Number: (850) 922-5864
Agency: Florida Department of Children and Families
Public Information Number: (850) 488-4855

Georgia

Agency: Georgia Department of Community Health
Public Information Number: (404) 657-0625
Agency: Georgia Department of Human Resources
Public Information Number: (404) 656-4937

Guam

Agency: Guam Department of Public Health and Social Services
Public Information Number: (671) 735-7101

Hawaii

Agency: Hawaii Department of Human Services
Public Information Number: (808) 586-4888

Idaho

Agency: Idaho Department of Health and Welfare
Public Information Number: (208) 334-0668

Illinois

Agency: Illinois Department of Children and Family Services
Public Information Number: (312) 814-6800
Agency: Illinois Department of Human Services
Public Information Number: (217) 557-1564
Agency: Illinois Department of Public Aid
Public Information Number: (217) 782-3458

Indiana

Agency: Indiana Family and Social Services Administration
Public Information Number: (317) 233-4453

Iowa

Agency: Iowa Department of Human Services
Public Information Number: (515) 281-4848

Kansas

Agency: Kansas Department of Social and Rehabilitation Services
Public Information Number: (785) 296-3271

Kentucky

Agency: Kentucky Cabinet for Health and Family Services
Public Information Number: (502) 564-6786

Louisiana

Agency: Louisiana Department of Health and Hospitals
Public Information Number: (225) 342-1532
Agency: Louisiana Department of Social Services
Public Information Number: (225) 342-6700

Maine

Agency: Maine Department of Health and Human Services
Public Information Number: (207) 287-3707

Maryland

Agency: Maryland Department of Health and Mental Hygiene
Public Information Number: (410) 767-6490
Agency: Maryland Department of Human Resources
Public Information Number: (410) 767-7758

Massachusetts

Agency: Massachusetts Executive Office of Health and Human Services (EOHHS)
Public Information Number: (617) 727-6077
Agency: Massachusetts EOHHS—Department of Social Services
Public Information Number: (617) 748-2353
Agency: Massachusetts EOHHS—Department of Transitional Assistance
Public Information Number: (617) 348-8402
Agency: Massachusetts EOHHS—Division of Medical Assistance
Public Information Number: (617) 210-5435

Michigan

Agency: Michigan Department of Community Health
Public Information Number: (517) 241-2112
Agency: Michigan Family Independence Agency
Public Information Number: (517) 373-7394

Minnesota

Agency: Minnesota Department of Human Services
Public Information Number: (651) 297-7717

Mississippi

Agency: Mississippi Department of Human Services
Public Information Number: (601) 359-9662
Agency: Mississippi Division of Medicaid, Office of the Governor
Public Information Number: (601) 359-6050

Missouri

Agency: Missouri Department of Social Services
Public Information Number: (573) 751-3770

Montana

Agency: Montana Department of Public Health and Human Services
Public Information Number: (406) 444-2596

New Mexico

Agency: New Mexico Children, Youth, and Families Department
Public Information Number: (505) 827-6984
Agency: New Mexico Human Services Department
Public Information Number: (505) 827-7781

New York

Agency: Office of Children and Family Services
Public Information Number: (518) 473-7793
Agency: Office of Temporary and Disability Assistance
Public Information Number: (518) 474-9516
Agency: New York State Department of Health
Public Information Number: (518) 474-7354
Agency: New York State Department of Labor
Public Information Number: (518) 457-5519

North Carolina

Agency: North Carolina Department of Health and Human Services
Public Information Number: (919) 733-9190

North Dakota

Agency: North Dakota Department of Human Services
Public Information Number: (701) 328-4933

Amira C. Tame, A.C.C.

Ohio

Agency: Ohio Department of Job and Family Services
Public Information Number: (614) 466-6650
Oklahoma
Agency: Oklahoma Department of Human Services
Public Information Number: (405) 521-3027
Agency: Oklahoma Health Care Authority
Public Information Number: (405) 522-5484

Oregon

Agency: Oregon Department of Human Services
Public Information Number: (503) 945-5652

Pennsylvania

Agency: Pennsylvania Department of Public Welfare
Public Information Number: (717) 787-4592

Puerto Rico

Agency: Puerto Rico Department of the Family
Public Information Number: (787) 294-4942
Agency: Puerto Rico Department of Health
Public Information Number: (787) 274-7676

Rhode Island

Agency: Rhode Island Department of Children, Youth, and Families
Public Information Number: (401) 528-3575
Agency: Rhode Island Department of Human Services
Public Information Number: (401) 462-6260

South Carolina

Agency: South Carolina Department of Health and Human Services
Public Information Number: (803) 898-2865
Agency: South Carolina Department of Social Services
Public Information Number: (803) 898-7602

South Dakota

Agency: South Dakota Department of Social Services
Public Information Number: (605) 773-3165

Tennessee

Agency: Tennessee Department of Children's Services
Public Information Number: (615) 741-9192
Agency: Tennessee Department of Finance and Administration
Public Information Number: (615) 741-2401
Agency: Tennessee Department of Health
Public Information Number: (615) 741-3111
Agency: Tennessee Department of Human Services
Public Information Number: (615) 313-4707

Texas

Agency: Texas Department of Aging and Disability Services
Public Information Number: (512) 438-3280
Agency: Texas Department of Family and Protective Services
Public Information Number: (512) 438-4384
Agency: Texas Health and Human Services Commission

Public Information Number: (512) 424-6951
Program Eligibility Verification Number: (512) 438-3280
Agency: Texas Workforce Commission
Public Information Number: (512) 463-2222

Utah

Agency: Utah Department of Health
Public Information Number: (801) 538-6339
Agency: Utah Department of Human Services

Dementia / Alzheimer's-Specific Sites

Administration on Aging, Alzheimer's Resource Room *http://www.aoa.gov/alz/*
From the Department of Health & Human Services' Administration on Aging, this link goes directly to the department's resources for professionals and the public regarding Alzheimer's. The public can get information on caregiving, health maintenance, working with physicians and more about the disease. Professionals can access assessment tools, disease management guidelines, training materials and more.

Alzheimer's Association *www.alz.org*
The Alzheimer's Association is a national volunteer health organization composed of a national network of chapters. It offers education, research grants and support for people with Alzheimer's, their caregivers and families. Its Web site is devoted to the activities of its mission and offers information for professionals, caregivers, patients and the media.

Alzheimer's Disease Cooperative Study
http://www-alz.ucsd.edu/
Alzheimer's Disease Cooperative Study (ADCS) is a sponsored consortium from the National Institute of Aging and the University of San Diego. Its goal is to further all activities related to clinical research in the area of Alzheimer's. Its Web site describes its activities and offers links to information on clinical trials, clinical sites and more.

Alzheimer's Disease Education and Referral (ADEAR) *http://www.alzheimers.org/*
The Alzheimer's Disease Education and Referral (ADEAR) Center's Web site is a service of the NIH's National Institute on Aging. Scroll down the main page to access information to research, clinical trials and more.

Alzheimer Research Forum
www.alzforum.org
The Alzheimer Research Forum is an online scientific community dedicated to developing treatments and preventions for Alzheimer's disease. It provides resources, news, compendia and discussion on its Web site.

ALZwell, Caregiver Page
www.alzwell.com
A resource for caregivers, ALZwell offers news, frequently asked questions, bookshelf, eldercare topics, dementia care topics and more. Caregivers can access a learning education series, which include resource guides, a pharmacy discount program, and audio and videocassettes.

The Cognitive Neurology and Alzheimer's Disease Center *http://www.brain.nwu.edu/*
The Cognitive Neurology and Alzheimer's Disease Center, or CN-ADC, is located in Chicago and conducts research to discover how the brain coordinates mental functions such as memory, language, attention and emotion. It treats patients and trains professionals in this area. The Web site describes the center's various projects, research and educational opportunities.

Dementia.com *www.dementia.com*
Dementia.com offers consumers and professionals information about dementia and Alzheimer's.
Healthcare professionals are required to register to access portions of the site.

Dementia, Mental Health in Later Life *www.mhilli.org/dementia*
From the U.K.-based Mental Health Foundation, this link takes users directly to the foundation's information on dementia. It offers discussion forums for various audiences, including professionals and caregivers. It also features access to various research projects being conducted in the area of dementia, as well as results of completed studies and projects.

Doctor's Guide to Alzheimer's Disease *http://www.docguide.com/news/content*
Visit the Doctor's Guide channel for Alzheimer's disease to read the latest medical news and alerts, Alzheimer's information, and to access discussion groups and newsgroups.

Dementia Research Group *http://dementia.ion.ucl.ac.uk*
Based at the National Hospital for Neurology & Neurosurgery in London, the Dementia Research Group conducts clinical trials in dementia, with a focus on Alzheimer's. It has more information on the genetic traits and psychology of dementia, and information on the clinical trials the hospital is conducting.

Elder Care Online *www.ec-online.net*
Elder Care Online is an online community that provides a message board on elder care, a newsletter and separate sections on elder care issues such as Alzheimer's, home care and more. The Web site also provides links to services and a bookstore.

Healing Well.com, Alzheimer's Disease Resource Center *www.healingwell.com/alzheimers*
Healing Well.com's Alzheimer's Disease Resource Center offers news and information culled from other Web sites. It also features online chat groups, a bookstore, a video center and more.

Mayo Clinic, Geriatric Medicine, Dementia Epidemiology *http://www.mayo.edu/geriatrics-rst/Dementia.I.html*
Geared toward professionals, this link goes directly to Mayo Clinic's comprehensive information on dementia epidemiology and includes diagnostic criteria for various dementias and risk factors.

Mayo Clinic.com, Alzheimer's Center *http://www.mayoclinic.com/findinformation/conditioncenters/centers.*

cfm?objectid=0007C524-3895-1B32-82D780C8D77A0000

The Mayo Clinic.com's Alzheimer's Center features news, articles, resources and information on the disease.

MedLine Plus *http://www.nlm.nih.gov/ medlineplus/dementia.html*
This link directs users to the National Library of Medicine and the National Institutes of Health reference site on dementia. It offers categories and links to other Web sites about dementia. Categories include clinical trials, news, coping and more.

The Merck Manual of Geriatrics, Dementia *http://www.merck.com/pubs/ mm_geriatrics/sec5/ch40.htm*
Taken directly from the manual, users can read about different dementias, diagnostic criteria, treatment issues and link to tables of supporting information.

Neurology Channel, Dementia *http:// ww.neurologychannel.com/dementia/*
Neurology Channel offers an overview of dementia, its causes, risks, symptoms, diagnosis and treatment information, which is geared toward the public.

REMINYLâ (galantamine HBr) Web Site *http://w.us.reminyl.com/*
From Janssen Pharmaceutica Products, L.P., this is an online information and support resource for caregivers, individuals who are concerned about Alzheimer's disease, and healthcare professionals. Full prescribing information is available.

Sharing Care™ *http://www.sharingcare. com/*
Sharing Care™ provides a free caregiver support program. Registered members have instant access through a personal home page to personalized information, relevant news specific to AD, valuable treatment tips for caregivers, and all the Sharing Care™ community support and resources.

The following are listings of additional recommended resources additional information on Alzheimer's disease.

The Alzheimer's Association has a network of more than 200 local chapters nationwide, providing programs and services to families and professionals within their communities. Support groups, telephone helplines, educational programs, publications and information about local services are available locally or through the association's national office:

Alzheimer's Association
919 North Michigan Ave., Suite 1000
Chicago, IL 60611-1676
(800) 272-3900 or (312) 335-8700
Fax (312) 335-1110
E-mail: info@alz.org or www.alz.org

Alzheimer's Support Websites
The following Web sites provide excellent information for laypeople on research developments, caregiving and support services for individuals and families coping with Alzheimer's disease:

The Alzheimer's Association
http://www.alz.org
Alzheimer's Association of Israel
http://www2.NetVision.net.il/~aai/

Alzheimer's Association (Australia)
http://www.span.com.au/span/alzheim.htm

Alzheimer's Association, Northern Virginia
Chapter
http://www.alz-nova.org/

Alzheimer's Association Victoria (Australia)
http://www.vicnet.net.au/alzheim/index.html

Alzheimer's Disease Education and Referral
Center, National Institute of Aging
http://www.cais.net/adear/

The Alzheimer's Disease Web Page
http://med-amsa.bu.edu/Alzheimer/home.html

Alzheimer Europe
http://www.alzheimer-europe.org

Alzheimer Page
http://biostat.wustl.edu/alzheimer/
Alzheimer Society of Canada
http://www.alzheimer.ca
Association of Family Carina for the
Demented Elderly, Japan
http://www2f.meshnet.or.jp/~boke/boke2.htm

Bedford Geriatric Research Education
Clinical Center, Bedford, MA

httlp://med-www.bu.edu/Alzheimer/home.html

The Cognitive Neurology and Alzheimer's
Disease Center, Northwestern University
Med School
http://www.brain.nwu.edu

The Dementia Web at The National
Hospital for Neurology and Neurosurgery
and The Institute of Neurology
http://dementia.ion.ucl.ac.uk/

Federazione Alzheimer Italia
http://www.geocities.com/HotSprings/1420/

Fundacion Alzheimer España
http://www.eurociber.es/solitel/alzheimer
Heather Hill Hospital, Health & Care
Center, Chardon, OH
http://www.heatherhill.com/
The Institute for Brain Aging and
Dementia, University of California
http://teri.bio.uci.edu/dement.html

List of all Alzheimer's Disease Centers,
National Institute of Aging
http://www.cais.com/adear/adcdir.html

Partners Program in Alzheimer's and Other
Neurodegenerative Diseases
http://www.partners.org/partners/alzheimers

National Institute of Mental Health
Alzheimer Disease Genetics Initiative
http://nimh.sratech.com/cgi

The University of Washington, Alzheimer's Disease Research Center
http://weber.u.washington.edu/~adrcweb/

Washington University—Alzheimer's Disease Research Ctr
http://www.biostat.wustl.edu/adrc/welcome.html

National Institute of Aging, News on Alzheimer's Disease
http://www.cais.com/adear/nianews.html
Transcripts on Alzheimer's Disease at Journal Graphics Home
http://www.tv-radio.com/~kelsy/topics/alzheime.htm
Idaho

Alzheimer's Information Resource Database

Alzheimer's Disease Education and Referral Center, National Institute on Aging

The Alzheimer's Disease Education and Referral (ADEAR) Center is a service of the federal government's National Institute on Aging (NIA), one of the National Institutes of Health.

National Institute of Mental Health, National Institutes of Health The National Institute of Mental Health (NIMH), a component of the National Institutes of Health, conducts and supports research that seeks to understand, treat, and prevent mental illness.

Neurological Disorders and Stroke, National Institutes of Health

The National Institute of Neurological Disorders and Stroke (NINDS) was originally established in 1950.

The NINDS conducts and supports research and research training on the causes, prevention, diagnosis of neurological disorders.
National Institute on Aging, National Institutes of Health The National Institute on Aging (NIA) was established in 1974 to conduct and support biomedical, social, and behavioral research and training relating to the aging process.

Agency for Healthcare Research and Quality

The Agency for Healthcare Research and Quality, formerly the Agency for Health Care Policy and Research, is the primary source of Federal support for research on problems.

Agency for Healthcare Research and Quality Publications Clearinghouse, Agency for Healthcare Research and Quality The Agency for Healthcare Research and Quality's *(formerly the Agency for Health Care Policy and Research)* publications cover such topics as medical treatment effectiveness and health care costs.

Alzheimer's Association

The Alzheimer's Association is a nonprofit organization founded in 1980 to heighten public awareness of this degenerative brain disorder, provide support for patients and their families.

Alzheimer's Disease Research Center

The Alzheimer's Disease Research Center (ADRC) is a program of research at the Johns Hopkins University School of Medicine. ADRC is supported by a major grant from the National Institute on Aging,

American Academy of Neurology

The American Academy of Neurology (AAN) is a professional society composed of neurologists and professionals in related fields who share a common goal of continued growth and development of the neurol

National Institute of Environmental Health Sciences, National Institutes of Health

Established in 1966, this Institute supports and conducts basic research focusing on the interaction between humans and potentially toxic or harmful agents in their environment.

After You Were Taken, Mother

After you were taken Mother I thought you would like to know what happened to me. Should I tell the truth, will you promise not to be mad at me? First of all, I wish every mother could live forever . . . because . . . . life is more fun when it's filled with love and peace. What a nice feeling it is when I call mom and she is there for me. It brings life back even when I don't feel good. When I see your smile it brightens up my day.

I have more and more to say about you. But today, Mother after you were taken, my eyes can't see the light. It feels like rain and darkness is in my way. I hear the wind. Sounds like it's mad at something. The trees and leaves are scattered everywhere, and the branches are split apart and covered with weeds. The birds and geese are flying out of control. They don't know which way to go. They are trying to find a safe place to survive. I see the lake and their waves hiding between the rocks and the sand is not in the way.

Here I am, no longer afraid. I lost my best friend, you, Mom. The love I got in my heart is no longer there. No sun, no warm heart to feel the heat. When I walk I need silence to learn new things. Things that that I am not aware of. I have to learn to touch and feel. Maybe it will help me learn how to trust again with no fear. I feel alone and cold. No one seems to care. I thought that someone would understand how I feel, and listen to everything I need to say. Mom, it's okay when I talk to you. I feel your presence, and my heart feels the warmth. Mom, nobody can ever give me love like you do.

Mom, everything that you and I used to do, we can't do again, because no one can take your place. I will always feel cold and I will walk and walk until you find someone to warm up my soul. Mom, can you tell me which way I need to go? I see clouds, but I can't tell what they are. Mom, I feel lonely. I don't even know if the flowers are for me. Maybe they will be my best friend to bring me warmth. Mom, I am still waiting to feel your touch or breath in my face or hear your voice to let me know where you are, because it's part of me. Mom, come visit me when you can and let me know you are here by feeling your soul.

Mom, do you want to know something? I still have the baby monitor in your room to hear you and run down when I know you need my help. Mom, guess what? It is still there for you. Now I watch the time and the days and nights and listen closely. It may be the time to visit your room and rest on your bed. My hope never dies. Someday I will hear your voice when the time is right and I'm no longer afraid. And I will say, Mom, please stay. Don't go away. Mother, I will always love you. When I die, I will see you there.

Your Loving Daughter (with a broken heart),

Amira

www.ingramcontent.com/pod-product-compliance
Lightning Source LLC
Chambersburg PA
CBHW031832170526
45157CB00001B/275